Zone Therapy Using Foot Massage

Astrid I. Goosmann-Legger

Zone Therapy Using Foot Massage

Translated from the Dutch by Tony Langham
and Plym Peters

with a foreword
by
Dr. A. M. Wesselius

SAFFRON WALDEN
THE C. W. DANIEL COMPANY LIMITED

First published in Great Britain by
The C. W. Daniel Company Limited
1 Church Path, Saffron Walden
Essex, CB10 1JP

Originally published in Holland
under the title, *Zone-Therapie dor Voetmassage*
by De Driehoek BV, Amsterdam

Reprinted 1988
Reprinted 1992

ISBN 0 85207 170 1

Designed by Tina Dutton
Production in association with
Book Production Consultants, Cambridge.
Typeset by Cambridge Photosetting Services in Bembo
Printed in Great Britain by
St Edmundsbury Press Ltd, Bury St Edmunds, Suffolk.

Contents

Foreword

Reflexology therapy is a form of manual therapy which makes use of the reflex points of the organs of the body, which can be found on the feet and ankles.

Even in ancient times, the Chinese knew about the reflex zones of the internal organs, which can be found over the entire surface of the body. This science has been applied for more than a thousand years – particularly in acupuncture – in order to influence the organs and organ systems.

All the organs appear to have their specific projection points on the feet, in the same way as they have been shown on the hands and ears. By means of carefully localised and measured amounts of pressure, it is possible to influence the way in which the organs function. This can have either a stimulating or a relaxing effect, depending on the amount of pressure exerted.

Conversely, organs which are temporarily or permanently "out of balance" can have an effect on the reflex zones which can express itself in visible changes, such as, for example, differences in colouration, swelling, tangible changes in body tissue such as softening or hardening of the tissues, and spontaneous pain or pain resulting from pressure. Thus the feet can play an important role, both in a diagnostic and a therapeutic capacity.

A thorough anatomical and physiological knowledge of the body and of the reflex zones is required to correctly evaluate the signs on the feet and to respond to them in a responsible fashion with a series of massage sessions.

This book clearly outlines what is possible and what is not in the field of reflexology.

The reader will gradually come to understand the important role that can be played by reflexology in the diagnosis and treatment of virtually the entire system.

Apart from writing about the positive effects, the author does not omit to indicate the limitations of the method, and points out the possibilities of combining reflexology with other disciplines, notably medical treatment.

At the same time, you will be surprised to find, as I was, when I first read this succinct book, how precisely the feet reflect the functioning of the human body.

But make no mistake – a great deal of skill, understanding, insight and experience is required to come to the straightforward conclusions which Astrid Goosmann seemingly produced without any effort.

The practice of reflexology should be learned under expert guidance.

Apart from this, your own enthusiasm for the subject, as well as the necessary knowledge of the structure and functions of the human body must be your guideline. In particular, those people who have massage in their fingertips, such as beauticians, physiotherapists, manual therapists, sports masseurs etc. may find that foot massage is a valuable addition to their knowledge.

In the field of medicine, reflexology can be an important addition in differential diagnosis.

Patients will certainly have to get used to the idea of taking off their socks and shoes when they come with stomach complaints or a painful shoulder. But after all, it's common practice now to treat a headache with suppositories.

Dr A. M. Wessalius

Introduction

In 1975 our college for beauticians in Rotterdam decided to include new forms of massage in the curriculum, in connection with the newly designed and experimental advanced course which we were in the process of setting up.

As the range of these courses was wider at that time in Germany than in the Netherlands, I went through their list of methods of massage and came across the reflex zone massage.

I enrolled and turned up on the first day of the course to find to my complete surprise that the massage in question was foot massage. This had not been my intention at all. After the first half of the course I returned to Holland rather disillusioned and extremely sceptical, and doubtful about returning for the second half.

However, I did return, from a feeling of duty and because I did not want to waste the money I had already spent. I found the other people on the course so enthusiastic about it that I was once again surprised.

What had they discovered that I had not? (I certainly hadn't discovered it, because the course had done nothing for me.) The least I could do was to start working, using the information I'd been given, and with a typically straightforward Dutch mentality I began to test out and practise this "magic" that I so distrusted.

That was the moment my own enthusiasm began.

I am writing this book deliberately because I have seen this pattern emerge in so many people: incredulity followed by scepticism and a feeling of distrust of all that airy-fairy stuff.

The reaction of people during my treatment of their feet awakened a sense of curiosity and surprise which has in no way diminished after many years of experience.

Though I had little faith, I increasingly have to acknowledge that our feet provide such an accurate reflection of what is happening in our body and our spirit, that I now feel confident about saying that feet are always right, even if there is not always a rational explanation for it.

Again and again I am surprised to be making this voyage of discovery on a pair of feet.

All over the world I have tried to make contact with people and their feet to find out more. I am quite aware that there is always more to learn, but my life is richer as a result and it is a professional method that I enjoy using in my career, with successful results.

However, a book can never be complete, and I am not attempting to be exhaustive. The thousand nuances which are discovered and experienced during many years of work can simply not be described in a book of this scope.

A good foundation course is a prerequisite, and a great deal of practice is needed to learn to make associations and relativise the language of the feet.

Part I

The background to foot massage

Possibilities and limitations

There are many ways of influencing a person's health. An important category of these methods is formed by a wide variety of massages.

This book deals only with the reflex zone massage of the feet, and an attempt is made to cover every aspect of this type of massage.

Specialist literature often attempts to establish a polarity between generally accepted western medicine and the alternative aspects of health care and the prevention of ill health. We consider that it is important to recognize the true value of any method that has proved itself to be effective, and not to reject any form of medicine out of hand. Even if methods of treatment have no rational explanation, it is wrong to deny their existence unless they have been shown to involve deceit, injury or to be worthless. Experience has shown that in the last case the method simply ceases to be used. Furthermore, there is no single method that can be the right one. A method which might be of great benefit to one person may not have the same results for another person.

To insist blindly on a single method of health care is very reprehensible and indicates a lack of ability to evaluate the relative worth of different possibilities. Thus health care should not be the exclusive domain of the medical profession.

On the other hand, sickness is a medical matter and should be dealt with by doctors, though the question may still arise whether a medical doctor should be the only person responsible for the patient's cure. Foot reflex massage is both a method of treatment and a form of therapy; it is used mainly by people who are not doctors. It should certainly never be used by anyone who is playing at being a doctor.

By studying the function of the foot reflexes, it is possible to determine the state of a person's health and to find out where there are disturbances in the function of his organs. The massage can:
– induce a state of relaxation;
– bring about emotional relief;
– improve the patient's general condition.

As soon as the foot reflexology indicates that the patient might be suffering from illness, or any serious impairment to health, it is absolutely essential to contact a doctor. Cooperation with the patient's own G.P. or with a specialist is vitally important for the patient if it is found that he benefits from this form of treatment.

In philosopy, man has always been an object of study as a single totality, and the distinction between the body and the soul has never been satisfactorily explained. We do not intend to go into this question here.

We simply assume the existence of both aspects and note that many different factors can have an influence. At the risk of stating the obvious, some of these factors are listed below at random:
– heredity
– the earth's gravity
– the movement of the sun, moon and stars
– the food we eat
– hormones
– the climate we live in
– the sleep we get or do not get
– pressures of society.

This list could be extended endlessly with factors which influence our well-being. Bearing this in mind, it would seem difficult and even extremely arrogant to choose a single therapeutic method as a panacea for every disturbance that can interfere with the human functions.

With regard to the importance of reflex foot massage, it has been shown that treatment of the foot reflexes can lead to:
– an increase in the dynamic force throughout the body and
– improvement in the circulation,
with a resulting
– increased output and output of matter and energy in the body;
– an adjustment of any imbalance in the material and spiritual equilibrium.

Origins of foot reflexology therapy

The American doctor, William Fitzgerald (1872–1942), is

considered as the founder of foot reflexology as it is known today.

Dr. Fitzgerald was an ear, nose and throat specialist. In his work and his lectures he contributed to a form of therapy which was used in China, India and by Indian tribes, five thousand years ago. At that time it was already known that using pressure points on the feet could relieve pain in the body. This method was also known in Europe by the sixteenth century.

At the beginning of this century Dr. Edwin F. Bowers and Dr. Fitzgerald wrote the book, *Zone Therapy*. Eunice Ingham, a masseuse who also came from the United States, was responsible for perfecting the technique of massage, and in a series of clear illustrations she projected the various parts on the body to places on the feet. Hanne Marquardt, from Germany, who started working with Eunice Ingham in 1967, has also done a great deal of important work. Her book, *Foot zone massage as therapy*,★ and her courses, have contributed to the international recognition of this specialised form of alternative medicine.

Finally, Doreen E. Bayley, from England, deserves to be mentioned for her book, *Reflexology Today*. This is an invaluable work for the more advanced reflexology therapist.

The place of foot reflexology in eastern medicine

It is not easy to isolate the foundations of reflexology. The fact that this therapy was used centuries before western civilisation does not necessarily mean that earlier civilisations had suitable theories to explain its effects.

The most suitable explanation in a current conceptual framework is Chinese Taoism. We are familiar with yoga, and the concepts of yin and yang are not entirely foreign to our ears. Tao is literally translated as "the way", and it is based on the idea that man should strive as far as possible to be at one with nature. Unlike the Chinese religion, which

★De Driehoek, Amsterdam 1982

Fig. 1 The zones of the body

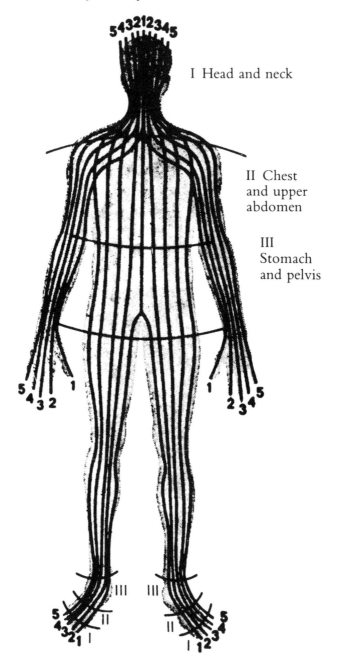

I Head and neck

II Chest
and upper
abdomen

III
Stomach
and pelvis

has two feet firmly on the ground, Taoism has a more magical and mystical slant. According to Taoism, the relationship between the universe and man can be demonstrated in many different ways. The totality of the universe can be rediscovered everywhere, projected into smaller totalities, like, for example, in man himself.

There are cosmic connections between the natural elements and the organs of the human body. Communication takes place between these elements and the organs along lines of energy which run throughout the body. Health depends on the unhampered interaction between the various projection areas, and treating this action is conducive to health and a method of combatting sickness.

The senses are the paramount projections and entry areas of the universe into the body. Iriscopy, auriculo (=ear) massage, and acupuncture are all founded on this principle, as well as reflexology. The latter is based on this because of the direct contact of the feet with the earth. (It is less applicable to the hands because with them there is no direct contact.) Because western medicine is familiar with, and accepts the effect of reflexes as reactions of the autonomic nervous system, the term "reflex lines" is used instead of "energy lines".

We will concern ourselves with the importance of the feet as a way of entering the organs via the reflex lines, and the following chapters will explain the sigificance of these for western or allopathic medicine.

Importance in western medicine

Western scientists, in this case doctors of medicine, do not easily accept reflexology. The fact that the therapy was known and used centuries before western civilisation does not necessarily mean that modern science can find a suitable theory to explain the effect.

Since the days of Ancient Greece there has been a scientific duel in western science between the idea that reality consists above and beyond the material environment perceived by our senses, and other theories based on a system of logic which can be determined by sensory experience.

No matter how many advances are made in western medical science, one incontrovertible fact remains: the arrogance about the omnipotence of rational thinking constantly seems to come up against a brick wall of new phenomena which cannot be simply explained logically. On the other hand, it is often the case that things which initially seemed inexplicable, turn out to have a logical explanation.

Reflexology falls between these two schools of thought. On the one hand, experience has shown that the massage is extremely effective. Results are facts, and even the most critical doctor could not deny this. On the other hand, there is no adequate explanation for massage being so effective, or why it is that certain parts of the body correspond with other parts of the body.

For many people in the west, something that has not been *proved* is not *true*. However, the problem is that it is no more possible to prove that it is not true. Thus all we can do is to continue the massage in the way that experience, based on results, has taught us.

What is reflexology

Every cell in our body has an electric charge, like everything around us. This electric charge is a form of energy and is influenced by our way of life. Just think of touching the door knob in a very dry room, stroking the cat, the crackle of a woollen jumper – the sparks can fly.

Sometimes the energy level is low and our motor system works slowly; sometimes the energy flies through us and we feel as though we can take on the whole world.

By treating various parts of the body in different ways with the hands, it is possible to influence these energy forms. That is what massage is. Obviously everyone is familiar with ordinary massage, concentrating on the muscles and the circulation of the blood; drainage aimed at the lymph circulation; pincements aimed at nerve ends etc. All these methods of treatment are based on West European philosophies.

However, Eastern philosophy is based on different principles. According to these principles there are energy lines running vertically, and more or less parallel, from head to foot (see fig. 1). The organism can be influenced at different points along these energy lines, e.g., at the energy points over the entire body, as in shiatsu; on the hands; on the ears, as in ear acupuncture; and on the feet. This last area of influence is the starting point for our form of massage.

The special aspect of our feet is that they are "earthed". We make contact with the earth through our feet. Just as a radio or television is affected by earthing it, the earth contact of our feet will help to reduce "interference" in our organism. In contrast with our feet, our hands have been

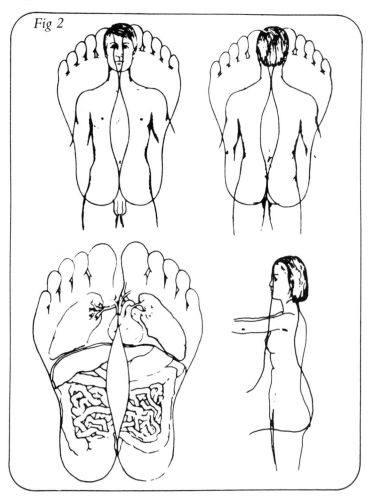

Fig 2

strongly cultivated. As a result, our feet are much more natural and "open" – they clearly reflect what the body wants to say. The masseur can gain a completely new insight from an extended observation of the feet. The book, *Stories the Feet can Tell*, by Eunice Ingham, means what the title says.

In fig. 2 the two bottom illustrations show a foot resting on its heel, and how the left and right-hand side of the body are revealed. This clearly demonstrates the principle: it couldn't be more clear, and in fact, it even shows where the various reflexes can be found on the feet.

Fig 3

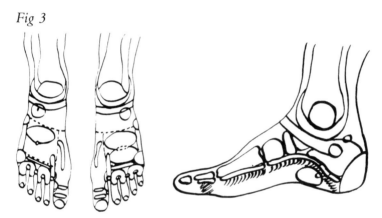

Now look at fig. 3. An imaginary line is drawn through the base joints of the toes, and a dividing line is drawn between the toes and the sole/instep. Basically this shows the division between the projection areas of the head and shoulders and the area below the shoulders. The chest area is projected exactly onto the zones of the metatarsals.

The arch of the foot represents the stomach area, and finally, the ankle area represents the pelvic area.

In principle this starting point will be used in the subject matter of the following chapters.

Man as a whole

When we have a complaint and go up to the doctor, the complaint is usually described in terms of pain, tiredness, aches etc. For example, we might have a stomach ache, be suffering from tiredness, or feel generally run down.

Normally this is followed by an anamnesis (a description of the complaint), an examination and medicine or medical advice. In most cases the therapy is aimed at the nature and location of the complaint. However, in cases of doubt about the isolated nature of the complaint, the doctor will usually check whether there might be a combination of causes, in a consultation session.

For a reflexology therapist it is often immediately apparent that the patient might be suffering from a number of different complaints, because he is able to recognise in miniature from observing and manipulating the feet, any organs that are not functioning properly. It is characteristic that though the patient may only mention one complaint, the therapist, after observing the feet, will often be able to ask the patient about complaints which he does not consider relevant himself, and therefore fails to mention.

Thus the feet can often indicate that there might be a connection between the complaints that have been mentioned, and others that have possibly not even been experienced. The following example, which took place about three years ago, is a good illustration of this.

A patient came to me with serious back pains, for which a doctor had given her tranquilisers and painkillers. There were no visible anatomical irregularities of any significance. Because I was extremely busy at the time, I treated her symptomatically. The pain decreased considerably, but a fortnight later she telephoned again because the pain had become worse than ever. Again I had to treat her on the basis of her symptoms because I had little time, but we made an appointment for a complete examination. During this session I came across a piece of "concrete" instead of a supple intestinal reflex. When I asked her about her bowel movements, she told me that by using laxatives, she was only able to move her bowels once a week. This concentration made her back rigid, so after this I concentrated on her intestines. After a few weeks she only had to come for ten minutes a week, and shortly afterwards her bowel movements had completely returned to normal and she was able to move her bowels every day without medication. Up to now the complaint has not returned.

The clear lesson to be learned from this is that man is a single whole, and the feet are a corresponding projected whole. For every complaint the therapist must therefore examine the entire feet to find out where the balance is disturbed. It is only when this has been done that it is possible to judge whether treating just a few reflexes is all that is needed.

A combination of possibilities

As the introduction stated, reflexology is not the only alternative form of medicine. There are many other forms using different starting points, but they all have a single common objective: to keep people healthy or to restore them to health.

It is quite possible to combine reflexology with one or more other forms of medicine including, for example, acupuncture, auriculotherapy (ear massage), manual therapy, homeopathy, hydrotherapy, iriscopy (more of a diagnostic method), herbal remedies, massages, food therapies and yoga.

These are only some of the best known therapies, some of which can be further sub-divided into specialised forms. Obviously these are all in addition to allopathy, the treatment generally accepted in our society and practised in western medicine. Thus there are plenty of possible combinations. Of course, all these different methods cannot be applied together. Too much stimulation from too many different directions can have a bad effect.

Part II

What feet reveal

What feet reveal

By observing a pair of feet without looking at the rest of the patient it is possible to gain an impression of his physical build: short, broad, thin, muscular, stout, sturdy or weak.

In many cases it is possible to recognise some of the probable problem areas in the body even at this early stage. When the feet are treated there are a number of factors which deserve special attention before starting on the massage. These factors are:

- What do the feet show?
- How do the feet feel?
- How do the feet smell?

What do the feet show?

Why is it so important to look at feet? Does the foot have a fallen arch? Is there something striking about the toe joint? Perhaps the metatarsals are too long or the heel is at an angle. All sorts of anatomical features may strike you. People with raised arches have hollow backs. It can be confusing if the arch of the foot is covered with tissue, but by feeling along the bony edges it is possible to find the true shape of the bones and any peculiarities.

Hard skin on the feet is another phenomenon that can be very revealing. Virtually all feet have some callouses as a form of natural protection. However, when the callouses are thicker in certain places or thicker than normal, or grow back quickly after a pedicure, it is possible to find out on which reflex this rapid growth is taking, and this reflex can then be considered to be *out of balance.*

It is commonly believed that callouses can only be caused by pressure from outside. However, this is only true when an abnormal external pressure leads to the reaction to form callouses. When there is a greater formation of callouses in a particular place, with or without external pressure, it is possible that the reflex is out of balance, and in this case the cause is inside the body. When there are corns, it is important to find out on which reflex the corns are situated.

There are different colours in the skin of the feet, which

may be red, white, purple, yellow or pink. The colours may differ from place to place on the foot. When they are bright red this means that there is too much blood passing through the corresponding reflexes. White is an indication of poor circulation, and purple indicates congestion. In the case of oedema or varicose veins, the exact location is also important.

Dry flakes of skin on the surface of a foot show that the corresponding area is lacking in energy. This means there is a disruption in the flow of energy. Cracks in the skin of the heels or between the toes are also very common.

During one course I once softly massaged chilblains. When I saw the patient a week later, the redness had disappeared and it never returned. I cannot think of any explanation for this, but it's not always necessary to explain things. In fact the awful aspect of many views on the influences of body and mind is that they always require an explanation. However, without an explanation, experience can often show what treatment should be used in order to achieve good results.

Patches of pigmentation are often found on parts of the foot with a predisposition towards these. One of my patients had a pigmentation mark on the point of the foot corresponding to the stomach. She had already told me that she suffered from asthma. When I asked her whether she had any other physical complaints, she told me she suffered from stomach pains. This had already been revealed by the pigmentation mark. The fact that she had had this mark from birth indicated that the stomach reflex formed a weak spot in her constitution. In the case of temporary ailments, discolouration of the skin sometimes takes place, but this may gradually disappear after treatment. For example, oedema, i.e., swelling of the ankles near the Achilles tendon, and on the upper side of the foot, may be caused by a malfunction of the heart, kidneys and the glands which produce internal secretions. Obviously it is necessary to distinguish between wet and fatty cushions.

How do the feet feel?

The first thing to feel is the temperature of the foot. It is not a good idea to wash the feet with hot or cold water before treatment because the correct temperature is lost. A cold foot can be fresh and cool, but it may also be chilly. A warm foot can be comfortably warm, but it can also be red hot. The foot may be damp with perspiration, clammy, varying from damp to wet. The more waste matter the body retains, the more the foot will perspire. In reflexology this can be interpreted as the body asking for a spring cleaning *through the foot*.

Tension can also be felt. This can be strong, with a good tension, or it can be weak. The flesh of the foot indicates the state of the tension in the corresponding reflex area. Local rigidity in the foot really belongs to the treatment because the reflexes where these rigid areas are found are important.

How do the feet smell?

Smelling the feet often leads to a few grimaces amongst people doing a reflexology course. However, it is important to consider the smell of the feet when giving treatment. There are basically two distinct types of smell:

The old cheese smell, which accompanies a large quantity of waste matter.

An acetone smell. When this smell predominates, the urinary system is involved.

External influences on the feet

It is best to treat feet in the morning, particularly when it is the first session of a course of treatment.

A. The feet have not been taxed and are not too tired, so that they present a more accurate picture. After standing in a shop all day long, or walking a number of miles, the reflexes react to tiredness caused by external factors and it is no longer possible to test the reactions of the reflexes correctly. This would give an incorrect picture.

B. Poor footwear, such as pointed shoes or high-heeled shoes etc., influence the reflexes and can eventually cause permanent damage to the body. Obviously this depends to a large extent on the resistance within the body.

C. Any traumatic external injuries, e.g., a cut or a sprain, will distort the reactions.

D. Deformities of the foot can give a distorted picture of the position of the reflexes on the foot.

If part of the leg has been amputated, it is possible to treat the amputated stump, though it is no longer possible to locate the reflexes. It would be better to concentrate on massaging the other foot and the reflexes on the hands and ears. It is possible to treat so-called "phantom pains" in this way.

Preventative effects of reflexology

Feet can give an indication of any imbalance in the body well in advance, and may react for a long while after a patient declares that he has been cured of his complaint. Because of this fact it is often possible to prevent the occurrence of many complaints.

Usually the patient seeks treatment because he has a complaint. However, a layman can take an interest in his feet, learn the language they speak, and if he takes the trouble to have treatment, he may spare himself many problems later on. Although I know this, I always wonder whether my feet are speaking the right language, and time and time again I have to admit that I have been unnecessarily sceptical.

Once I had a pain in my right foot, and when I looked to see which reflex was hurting, it was the bladder, the reflex of which is situated on the inside of the feet. When I pressed the reflexes, they hurt on both sides. I deliberately did nothing about it because I had no other complaint. Three days later I had an infection of the bladder, which I then treated.

A patient told me during an ordinary massage session that she was not sleeping with her husband because he had a terrible throat infection. On her feet I felt the throat reflex area, and it was very painful. By the following day she had also caught the throat infection.

Whenever I treat a man over forty years old, I always

examine the prostate area, without mentioning it. In this way it is possible to trace malfunctions which might cause grave problems later, and which can be treated at an early stage. It is better to prevent problems than to be forced to cure them later, a course which might even involve an operation.

Part III

The massage itself

The relationship between the patient and the therapist

Whenever a patient comes to see me, I put out my "feelers". This is both important and risky.

It is important because it enables me to register a number of facts which can help me in the examination, the diagnosis and the treatment.

It is risky because I must take care not to pigeon-hole the patient and draw premature conclusions.

How does a person present himself? Exuberant, quiet, despondent, controlled, untidy, dishevelled, heavily made up, or wearing too much jewellery? Does the patient dwell on his complaint in great detail, wallow in self-pity, or minimise all of his problems? Above all, I notice the expression in the patient's eyes: the lustre, the wetness, and the hard or soft expression. Eyes reveal many things.

At a course in the east of Holland I met a participant whose vision had deteriorated considerably over the years. Her optician was not able to discover the cause, but considering the progression of the condition, he had warned her that she would probably be blind within two years. An examination of the eye reflexes did not reveal anything regarding the pathology of the eyes. This surprised me so much that I took her to one side and talked to her. Her eyes were full of such terrible fear that I wanted to try and find out more about it. I didn't want to know where her fear stemmed from, but I wanted her to tell me how she felt. As a result of this conversation she was referred to a psychotherapist. After six months her optician declared that she had made unbelievable progress.

In treating the feet it is also important to constantly bear in mind the whole nature of the human being and his body. Psycho-somatic complaints are very often not suitable for reflexology, although treatment can often lead to an improvement in the physical condition by breaking through a vicious circle and stimulating a better psychic well-being.

The reflexologist must be able to admit to his inability to help a patient, and should then refer the patient to someone who can do more for him. The therapist can get a great deal of support from a close relationship with a patient which is based on an involvement with him or her. It is important to care for people, but it is just as important for the therapist to realise his own limitations and not to overestimate his abilities. If he feels dislike for a particular patient, for whatever reason, it is no good concealing this dislike behind a professional facade; the therapist should simply break off the relationship.

Speed, rhythm and depth of massage

The speed, rhythm and depth of massage are learned from experience, and learning to feel what is required. This does not mean that there are no general guidelines which can be listed and learned.

First the speed of the massage. This should be adapted to the person being treated. A nervous personality does not benefit from a high speed; the massage should be restful, so that the patient feels the benefit of it. Conversely a slow and listless patient will respond well to a more energetic form of massage.

The rhythm is concerned with the regularity of the massage. However, when a therapist is massaging a pair of feet, he will come across reflex zones which react with certain degrees of pain, where he will have to apply friction for longer periods of time.

In modern society more and more people wanting massage suffer from tension. If the therapist concentrates on relaxing the patient, subsequent sessions are extremely effective.

First, all the reflexes are massaged quietly and not too deeply, without paying any extra attention to the painful reflexes and using a steady rhythm, a sort of cadence in which it is important not to fall asleep.

The depth of the massage is quite evident, and should be as deep as the patient can endure. The patient must be able to feel the massage clearly, but the pain threshold should not be exceeded.

If it becomes immediately apparent that virtually anything is painful, this means that the massage is too heavy for the patient and it is necessary to reduce the pressure everywhere. However, if the patient can bear it, it is alright to apply pressure with the thumbs right down to the bone. There are some patients who feel pain as soon as the skin is touched with a finger. This seems incredible until you experience it yourself. After a while the correct treatment is learned, and the right speed, rhythm and pressure are automatically found.

The technique and procedure of the foot massage

Eunice Ingham treated the reflexes by employing a kind of "friction". She moved the fingers as though she was trying to pulverise grains of sugar, pushing the fingers a little deeper each time.

Hanne Marquardt uses a method which can best be described as "going for a walk". She places the thumb parallel to the area of skin to be treated, and then moves the thumb across it until it makes an angle of about 45°. The advantage of this rolling movement is that it massages the tissue and the final deep pressure of the thumb provides the real reflex stimulus.

In the course of my practice I have learned to value both techniques and to combine them. Walking the thumb has an ebb and flow effect, building up to a high point and then ebbing away. This rhythm in itself has a very relaxing effect. However, the problem of this technique is that learners are inclined to pull on the skin when the thumb has reached its deepest point. They seem to pull the nail under the joint of the thumb, which means that the pressure is not applied in depth, and that the skin is being pulled rather superficially.

The best method is to "take a walk" through the foot, and apply friction for some time, whenever pain or hard areas are encountered.

During massage it is good to have complete contact with the feet, using both hands, though without pinching them. The patient should be free to pull his foot away and should not have the feeling that his foot is stuck.

With regard to the order followed during massage, it is obviously important not to move around completely at random. It is possible to introduce a clear system following this procedure. In general, the therapist works on both feet consecutively on the same reflex area. For example, when the reflexes of the head are being treated, this is done on the two feet consecutively and it is not advisable to move on then to the pelvic reflexes and then the heart reflex.

There is a sort of to and fro movement in the massage, moving gradually from the toe reflexes, through the heel reflexes and then on to the lateral and medial reflexes, to end up with the treatment of the instep. It is perfectly possible to build up one's own order, but this should be based on a system learned from experience.

Pain during treatment

A distinction is made between various sorts of pain. A question that recurs frequently is: "Where should I feel pain during treatment? In my body, or in my feet?" Normally the pain is felt in the feet in the place of the painful reflex zone. However, it is very common to experience feelings on the body or to feel a glow of warmth in certain areas of the body.

During a course I massaged the feet of a student in the area corresponding to the spine, where she had a slipped disc. She told me that she suddenly felt a sensation of warmth in this spot on her back. When we looked at her back, we saw that it had reddened in that place. In a healthy person, someone who is in equilibrium, reflexology massage is experienced as a pleasant relaxed feeling. Every painful feeling can be described as one of three types:

1. Beneficial pain. This pain is best described as the feeling which is experienced when a stiff muscle is very softly and carefully eased.
2. A sharp pain. This pain can be described as the feeling which is experienced when the tissue is treated with a sharp object. It is a cutting pain. On the feet it is often felt in acute cases, or along nerve lines (e.g., on the sides of the toes).
3. Bruising pains. This sort of pain is best described as pressure on a bruise. It is a dull and painful ache, which is experienced in chronic cases.

Indications and counter-indications

No form of massage, including reflexology massage, should be practised when the patient has a temperature. The body is already fighting and does not require any extra burdens.

A severe inflammation or physical trauma should be dealt with by a doctor, and in cases of doubt, he should see the patient first.

A rudimentary tissue, e.g., an extra tooth, or a foreign body in the tissue, invariably becomes active and can start to move. If this movement occurs close to vital organs, e.g., in the breast or stomach, this can have serious consequences. For pieces of the roots of teeth that have remained after the teeth themselves have been extracted, this movement can produce excellent results, and they will undoubtedly come out.

For this reason reflexology therapy is also counter-indicated if the patient if the patient has thrombosis or is fitted with an i.u.d.

Obviously questions also arise with regard to serious illnesses, and there is also the familiar controversial question of massage in the case of cancer. One view holds that treatment is certainly possible. However, cancer means that a number of cells have given up being part of the body and are growing at the expense of the healthy cells.

A woman I knew who had had a mastectomy in hospital, asked me to treat her with reflexology therapy. Her own doctor had agreed. Though I was extremely sorry, I felt I had to refuse. Shortly afterwards she developed metastases. How would I have felt if I had treated her? However, later on I did treat her in the final stages of her illness in order to alleviate the pain and help her sleep so that she was better able to cope with the progressive development of the cancer.

I believe that reflexology therapy should not be practised on cancer patients before the terminal stage. However, in many other serious diseases some of the symptoms can be treated very well.

For example, in ankylosing spondylitis the progressive stiffening of the vertebrae can be slowed down.

In rheumatic patients massage can improve the condition and alleviate pain.

Reflexology treatment for heart conditions also deserves special attention. This will be discussed in the section devoted to this organ (see part V).

Direct and indirect approaches to the symptoms

During the initial stages, when one is learning to massage the feet, there is a tendency to massage the reflex belonging to the symptom. For a painful knee, the reflex of the foot is massaged; for a painful throat, the reflex of the throat. In many cases this is quite correct, but it often happens that the reflexes of the feet of a patient with a painful knee, do not indicate pain in that area, or that if the reflex is painful, repeated treatment does not reduce the pain or remove any pain in the area.

One of my patients complained of pain in her lower back and was massaged in the corresponding area without any obvious result. When I took her feet in my hands I noticed straightaway that she had a prolapsed bladder. I immediately referred her to her doctor. She had an operation, and the backache disappeared. This shows that the location of the complaint in the body is not necessarily the origin of it. In this case there was a causal relationship between origin and location.

There are three methods of treating the symptoms of a complaint:

1. There is a complaint in the body: the corresponding reflex is found and treated.

2. The causal relationship between a complaint and the location on the foot is sought; e.g., pains in the arm resulting from a problem in the neck vertebrae, pains in the knee caused by problems in the lower back or pelvic region. It is therefore necessary to ask what causes the complaint. Elsewhere I discuss the possible background to acne: hormonal, digestive, allergic or the result of stress. This is not a theoretical approach; the feet themselves provide the

answer. Changes and painful reactions indicate precisely where the problem lies.

3. The last possible method refers back to the beginning of the book, in which the vertical zones are described. If the above-mentioned points 1 and 2 do not provide any solution, it is worthwhile following the energy lines.

In our bodies, all the areas lying in a vertical energy line end in the feet in the same line as the reflexes of those areas. If the energy in this line of our body is blocked, other areas on the same line may not receive sufficient energy and this can lead to complaints there.

The most striking example I have experienced was a man with chronic pain in his right ear. By using the method described above, I found that the vertical part of the large intestine was extremely painful. After treating this part of the intestine for some time, the pain in the ear vanished. Once again the feet showed where the problem lay. It is only by knowing where the lines of energy run that it is possible to find the origin of a complaint by this method.

Number and frequency of treatments

In principle it is possible to continue treating a patient as long as there are reactions during and after the treatment. Some patients respond from the first session, while others require quite a few sessions before there is any reaction. On the whole, children and older people respond fairly quickly, while people in the prime of life usually respond rather more slowly. Therefore more care should be taken in treating children and older people.

I usually start a course of treatment with two sessions per week for the first three weeks, and then I discuss with the patient how the course of treatment should continue. If a patient is unable to come twice a week, it is possible to begin a course of treatment if he comes once a week. I gradually wind down the course of treatment by increasing the time between two consultations. There are patients who are in the habit of coming for a massage once a month to stimulate their physical functions.

Reactions during treatment

You cannot know or predict how a patient will respond during and after treatment. We will first discuss the possible responses during treatment. These may indicate the threshold of what the patient can endure. Every session of treatment is different, and what applies to one session may not necessarily be indicative for another session.

A. Perspiration of the hands. This often happens when a reflex zone is massaged which is prone to reaction at that moment. The massage can continue, but it is a good idea to reduce the pressure slightly.

B. Perspiration over greater areas of the body or over the entire body.
This is rather a violent reaction and it is advisable to stop the treatment and to be less intense at the following session.

C. A cold feeling starting in the limbs.
In this case it is also better to stop, in order to prevent:

D. Chattering of the teeth and the possible collapse of the circulation. This should never happen if the indications A, B, and C are properly observed.

You will understand why I'm always surprised when I read in magazines that anyone can do a foot massage and that people can massage each other's feet. In fact, an amateur can do considerable damage. An incorrect interpretation of what happens after the massage can also lead to the wrong conclusions, and this can give foot massage a bad reputation. If a patient starts to feel very uncomfortable during or after massage, even if you have been very careful, take the following steps:

Very quietly treat the solar plexus for a while and possibly the pituitary and the heart area. Cover the patient with something warm, especially his feet, and let him lie down for a while. Usually he will quickly recover.
A calm reaction from the therapist also has a reassuring effect and is therefore every bit as important.

If the treatment has come to a premature end because of the adverse reaction of the patient, it is possible to come to the conclusion that the treatment of this patient should no longer be continued. However, it is possible to treat the patient in particular areas, e.g., first the head zones, another time the chest area, and then a treatment of the digestive organs etc. Finally, larger areas can be treated during a single session.

Reactions after treatment

The first reaction after treatment is a relaxed and rather sleepy feeling. It is therefore extremely important to allow the patient to rest for a while, warmly wrapped up. If the patient has to drive home, it is particularly important to avoid the risk of his endangering other motorists.

A rest enhances the effect of the treatment and should certainly not be omitted.

The next day, or even a day or two after that, a number of different reactions may occur. These are all related to the removal of waste matter from the body. In some cases it almost seems as though the treatment has produced a negative reaction, but nothing could be further from the truth. One way in which the body gets rid of waste materials in what may seem to be a negative fashion, is that the complaint gets worse. This can be explained as follows:

1. In the air passages a persistent chill or an inflammation of the sinuses that leads to an excessive production of mucus and severe coughing, a cough that is becoming looser, or a runny nose, feel more serious and are more of a nuisance than a ticklish cough or a blocked-up nose. However, it is essential that the waste matter disappears.

2. Urination may increase. It can become more cloudy and can have a more pungent smell. This is particularly noticeable when there is a bladder infection.

3. A great deal of waste matter is removed through the intestines. Even if there are no physical complaints, it is often the case that stools will have a different composition

and will smell very unpleasant. In the intestines, waste materials left behind can accumulate, and good health depends on their removal.

4. In women, treatment can lead to increased vaginal discharge, a white mucus substance. This can last quite a long time, but as a reaction to foot massage it is a way of getting rid of waste matter.

I once gave foot massage to a girl who had menstrual problems. The problems disappeared, but a white discharge appeared. Her doctor prescribed medicines to treat this white discharge, whereupon the menstrual problems returned. She was simply preventing herself from getting rid of her waste matter in a natural way.

5. Waste matter is also removed through the skin. This can result in pustules or skin troubles. When I first meet cases of acne, I treat the feet to find out the origin of the acne; possibly the hormonal background (of puberty) may be the most important cause, or there might be digestive problems.

The patient might be under stress, and in a number of cases these factors are combined.

By combining foot massage with treating the skin and the acne itself, the chance of a cure is greater. However, in this case too, the first reaction might be a worsening of the complaint, which is later followed by a gradual and definite improvement.

Allergies will be discussed later under the treatment of the reflexes themselves.

6. Another reaction to massage is an increased temperature, which can rise as high as 38.5 °C. The temperature rises because of the increased body heat. However, obviously this is not the sort of fever that one has with an infection.

7. Infections which have not yet manifested themselves, e.g., in the teeth, can indicate that this part of the body is not in equilibrium by causing pain in the reflex areas. However, the body itself does not react with pain; only the reflex zones do. Obviously this is not a negative reaction because

preventative measures can be taken on the basis of this.

8. Past diseases which were not totally cured can become active again after massage, eventually finally to disappear.

9. One of the positive reactions which has no irritating side effects is that the patient sleeps more deeply and peacefully and finds it more easy to relax. A patient who often dreams, may find that he will sleep better for a few nights after the zones of the head have been treated.

10. The last reaction described above may be rather unexpected, but it is a more or less logical response. Obviously there is not only waste matter of a physical nature, but the patient may also be psychologically overburdened with waste matter. Who in our society can escape being occasionally stressed, even for prolonged periods. Actually this cathartic form could be classified under reactions during massage. However, as the effect usually lasts for a while, I include it in this section.

It is possible to provoke a psychological response which may be expressed in a number of different ways. Some patients get fits of the giggles, and occasionally the patient can give the impression that he has had quite a few drinks before his treatment session. However, this is merely a reaction to the massage. A more common reaction is for the patient to burst into tears, and it may not be possible to stop the flow – but really there is no need to do so.

Another reaction is that the patient may start to talk about his problems, sometimes in more detail than in retrospect he might have wished. Two important points should be remembered in this respect. The therapist must make it clear to the patient that he can feel safe to say anything and that this will be kept in complete confidence. The therapist should also assure the patient that he is familiar with human behaviour and that nothing the patient can say or do is "crazy", illogical or unusual.

On the other hand, the therapist must be very careful not to try and offer solutions. He is concerned with helping the patient to lose waste matter, and that is usually enough.

During the period when I first started practising I

remember a very cheerful patient who came to see me. I did not have much experience, and the patient seemed to be perfectly alright. During a treatment session she suddenly jumped out of her chair and ran to the toilet. A few minutes later she returned laughing with red and tearful eyes, behaving as though nothing was wrong. At a subsequent session she told me what was happening in her life. This seemed to me to be so serious that I immediately referred her to a specialist who was better able to help her. She accepted my advice, but before her appointment with the specialist came up, she telephoned me and said she would prefer to call it off. She felt that the treatment had helped her over an obstacle and that she could now cope with things on her own again. This is a clear example of changed behaviour after getting rid of psychological waste matter.

It is important to realise that these reactions do not all appear in one patient simultaneously. It is normal to expect one to three reactions after any session. The question often arises whether it might be advisable to prepare the patient in advance for the possible reactions. I do not recommend this for the following two reasons. First, it might alarm the patient, and secondly, the suggestion might have the effect of a self-fulfilling prophecy.

Usually I only tell the patient that he might feel as though he had a touch of flu the following day, and that he might have to go to the toilet more than he would normally. However, before the next session I always find out what the patient experienced after his previous session, and tell him that I can always be contacted by telephone if any problem arises. The most essential thing to remember if you come across any complaint of a serious nature – and even during treatment this might happen – is that you should strongly advise the patient to see his family doctor.

Aids to massage

The most sophisticated piece of equipment available for foot massage is our own hands. In addition to this unfailing tool, there are many aids available to help the hands: mats, cushions, bolsters, abacuses, wooden sticks etc. For a real expert these aids are not essential.

Obviously any part of our body that is untrained or over-used can start to become painful after a great deal of effort. This also applies to our thumbs, our hands and our arms after giving foot massage, but after the usual practice period, all this will start to function more easily. Obviously the muscles and nerves will protest in the beginning, but gradually all this disappears if one perseveres. The muscles of my hand are no better than anyone else's but they have never yet protested in all the years that I have been practising foot massage.

When you have learned to "touch" as well as to "feel" with the fingers, you will have acquired 90% of all you need to know about foot massage. You must learn to feel every slight nuance of the skin, muscles, nerves and bones, and this can never be replaced by any other artificial equipment. This wealth of information through the sense of touch determines the amount of massage needed, and again this cannot be replaced by any other artificial aid. There is no danger in giving too much massage. It is certainly true that the aids can give you warm feet, but this can be achieved with a warm bath, or by going for a walk, and after all, this is not the purpose of reflexology. And what could artificial aids do for the reflexes around the ankles, between the toes and on the instep. Absolutely nothing.

There is no aid that can properly massage the ankles and the instep, and an artificial aid is not able to gauge the fine nuances between the toes. There is only one medium to use for foot massage, and that is the hands.

Self-help

It is virtually impossible to give yourself a complete treatment of foot massage. Treatment takes a long time, and it is not possible to relax sufficiently to be able to profit to any real extent from this sort of complete massage. In addition, it is not possible to stand back, detach oneself, feel with the fingers in an objective way and assess the information the fingers have received.

However, it is possible to treat a limited number of reflexes, determined in advance, on your own feet, particularly when you have already been able to ascertain which reflexes are *out of balance*.

Sit down as comfortably as possible with some cushions under your back, preferably on your bed. Remember that your feet are in mirror image of feet you would be working on with a patient. One advantage is that your own feet are always close at hand.

The visually handicapped therapist

Although there are obviously many other handicaps than the loss of sight, it is important in this context to make an exception for this form of handicap. People who are partially sighted, or even completely blind, often have very strongly developed other senses: their sense of hearing, touch and smell may be far better than those of people who also have the sense of sight.

As the sense of touch is one of the most important senses for reflexology, I consider partially sighted people to be particularly suitable for this type of massage.

Part IV

The position of the reflexes

The tops of the thumbs are aligned along the reflex of the diaphragm. All the organs above the diaphragm in the body are also above this line in the foot.

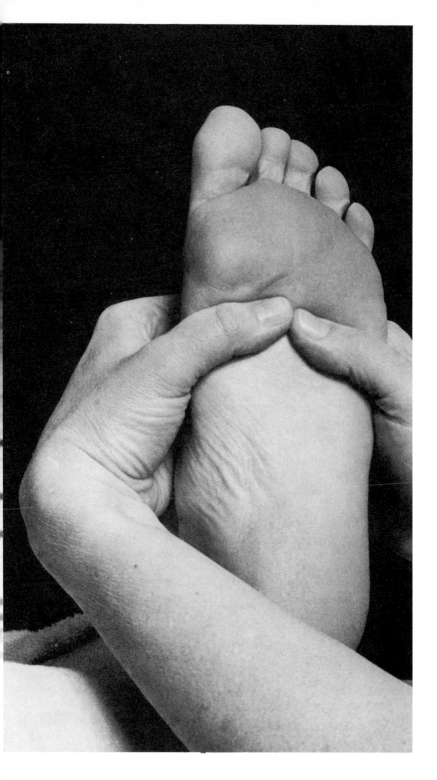

Where the two thumbs meet in the preceding photograph, along the line of the diaphragm, we find the solar plexus reflex, high up in the middle of the foot. This has a great influence on the automatic nervous system. All foot massage sessions should begin and end with the treatment of this reflex. The reflex is pressed in as the patient breathes in, and relaxed as he breathes out.

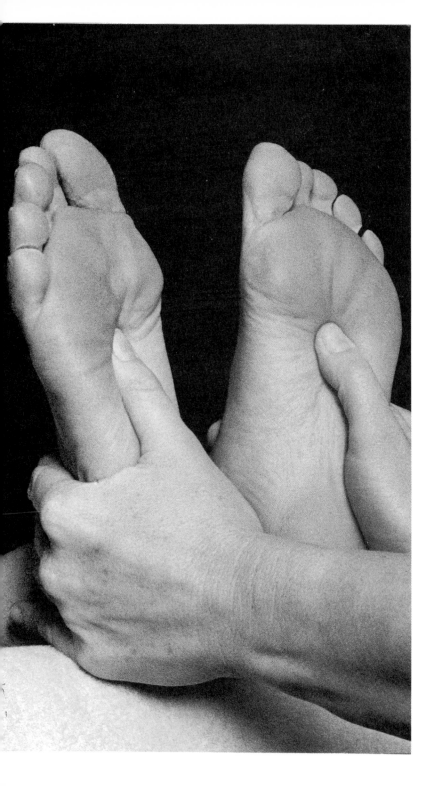

The position of the pituitary reflex. This reflex influences almost all the other glands with internal secretions, and if one or more of these is not functioning properly, it is advisable to massage the pituitary first, and then the gland concerned.

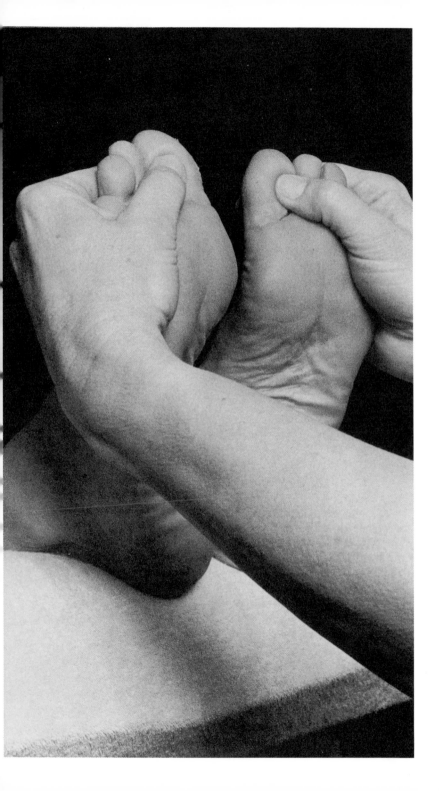

The reflexes of the neck muscles. Many neck pains are caused by tension in the neck muscles. It is also possible to relax the neck muscles to some extent by carefully rotating the big toe.

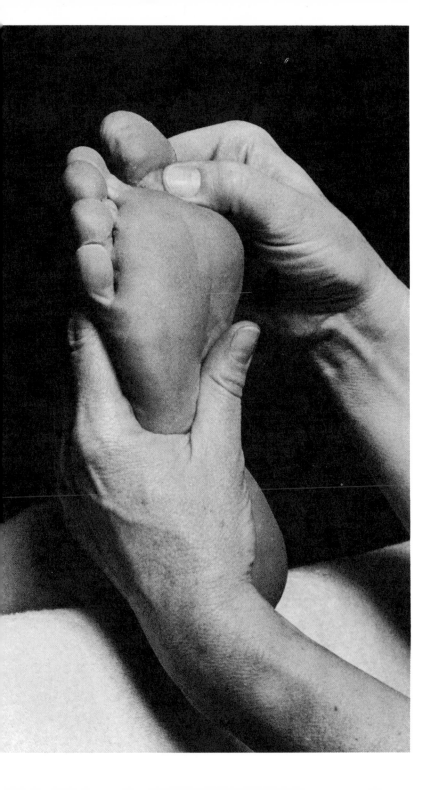

The position of the reflex of the *inner ear,* and the *semicircular canals*. This is the correct place to massage in connection with dizziness, car sickness or buzzing in the ears.

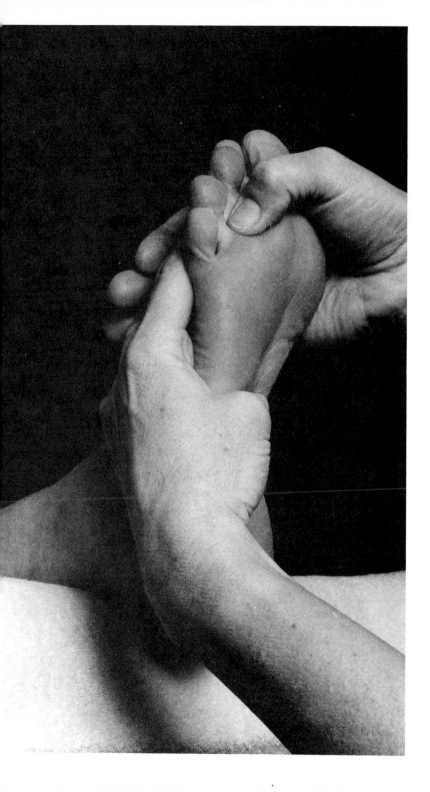

The position of the thyroid and the para-thyroid reflexes. Research into people with defective thyroids has shown that they can have an extreme reaction when this spot is massaged. There may also be a reaction in people who are very highly strung, even if there is no question of a malfunction of the thyroid.

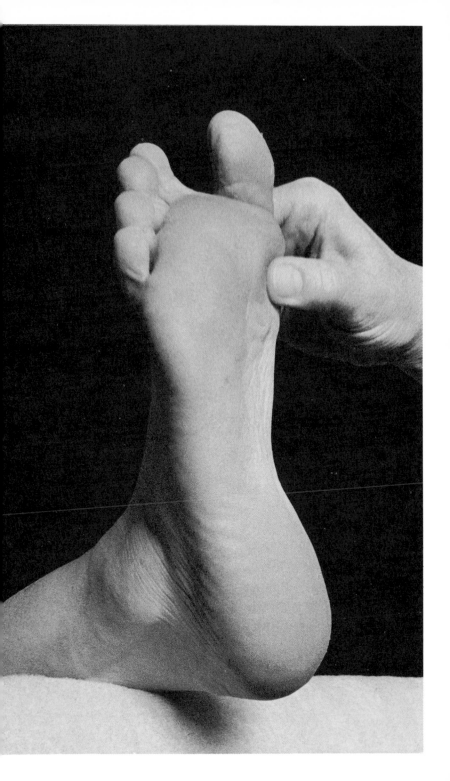

In this photograph the thumb is placed on the reflex of *shoulder joint*. This is surrounded by the tissue of the shoulder, and below the thumb lies the reflex of the lymph glands under the arms.

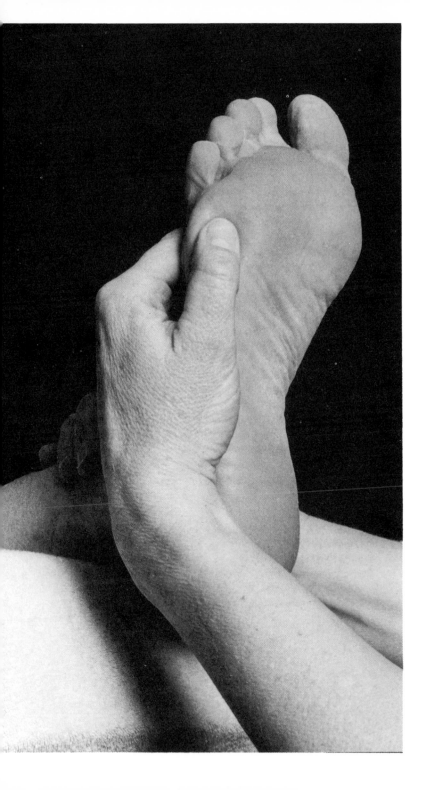

The lung reflex. The thumbs are placed on the area corresponding to the right lung. To the left and above this reflex are the reflexes of the shoulders, and below is the reflex of the diaphragm.

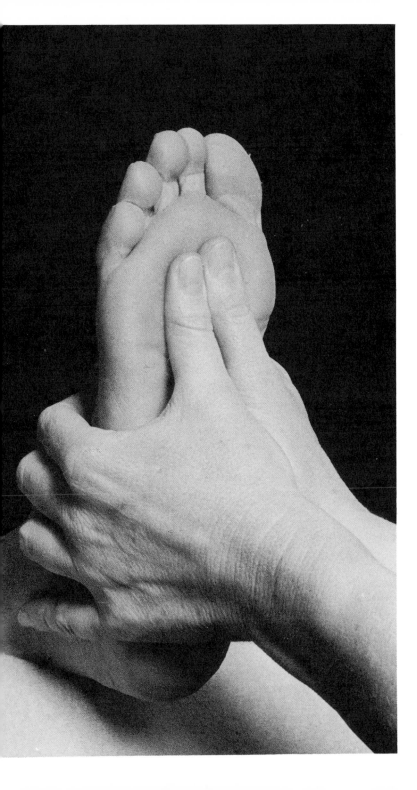

The two fingers are placed on the position of the *liver* reflex, which is situated immediately below the diaphragm reflex on the right foot. This reflex continues down towards the heel as far as the protruding fifth metatarsal on the outside of the foot.

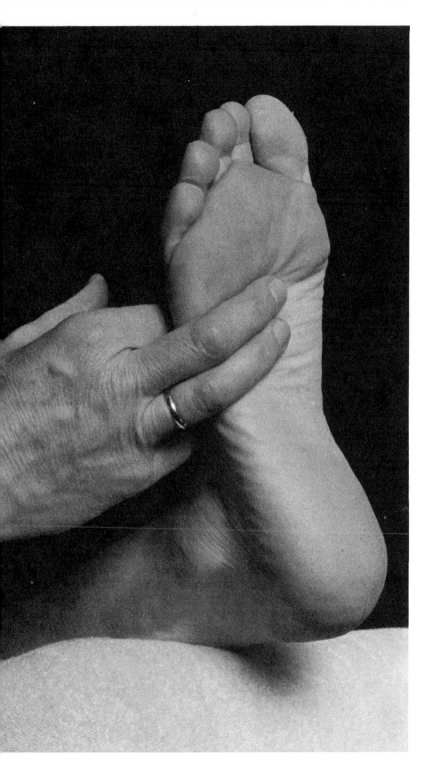

Within the liver area described in the previous photograph, lies the *gall bladder* reflex. Using the right thumb, the gall bladder can be clearly felt on the perpendicular line beginning between the third and fourth toe, where it crosses the liver.

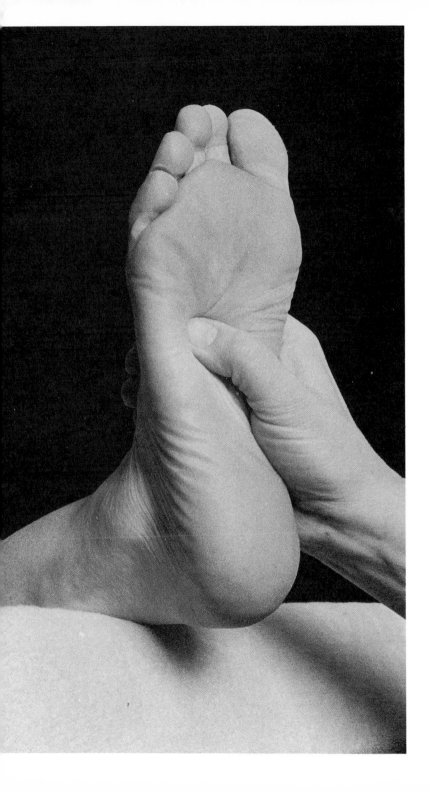

The reflex area of the *heart* lies on the left foot between the two thumbs. This reflex can be painful when (too much) pressure is used, and this is a warning sign when it is overburdened.

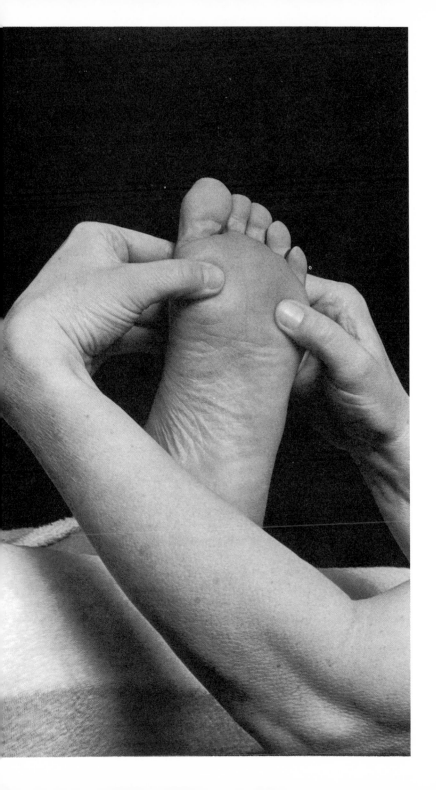

The *spleen* reflex lies under the upper reflex of the thumb. This reflex responds strongly in the case of particular infectious diseases, inflammations and great physical tiredness.

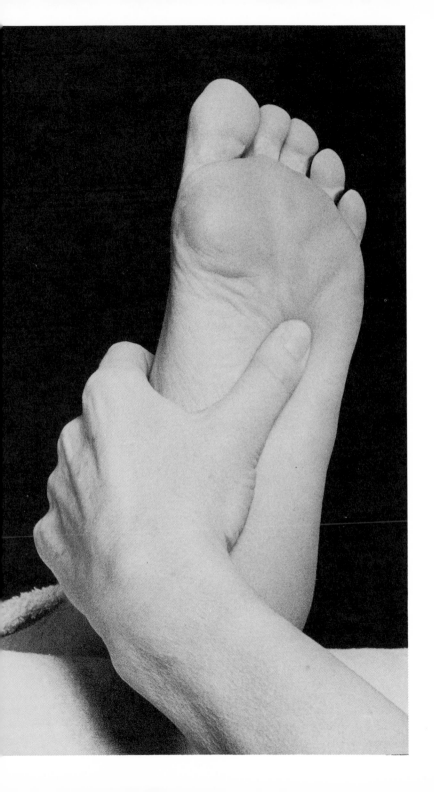

The reflex of the pyloric sphincter. The photograph showing the thyroid clearly shows the localised swelling which indicates that the pyloric sphincter is out of balance. This reflex responds clearly to tension. In fact, a number of the photographs show the reactions to certain reflexes; here, tension is revealed by the rigid position of the toes.

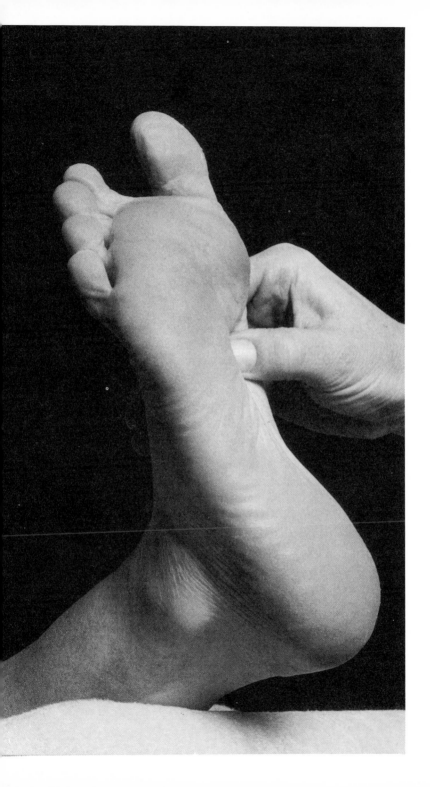

From the top of the thumb three-quarters of the thumb covers the area of the reflex of the *pancreas*. This area also contains the reflex of the *Islets of Langerhans*.

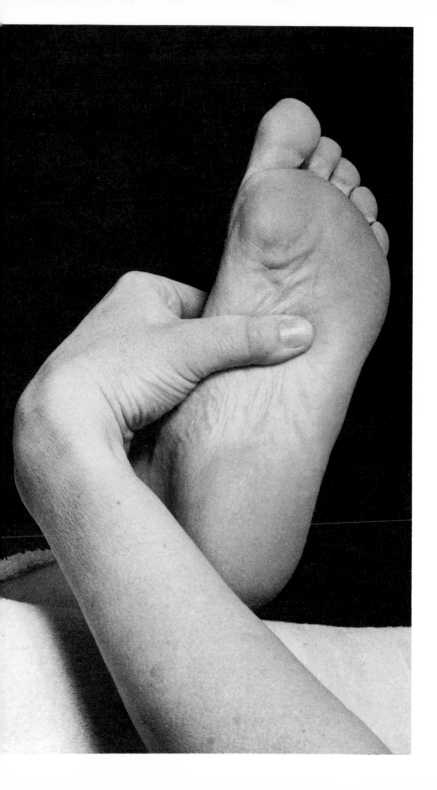

In this photograph the thumb is placed on the central area of the *small intestine* on the left foot. This reflex is virtually entirely surrounded by the reflex of the large intestine (see next photograph).

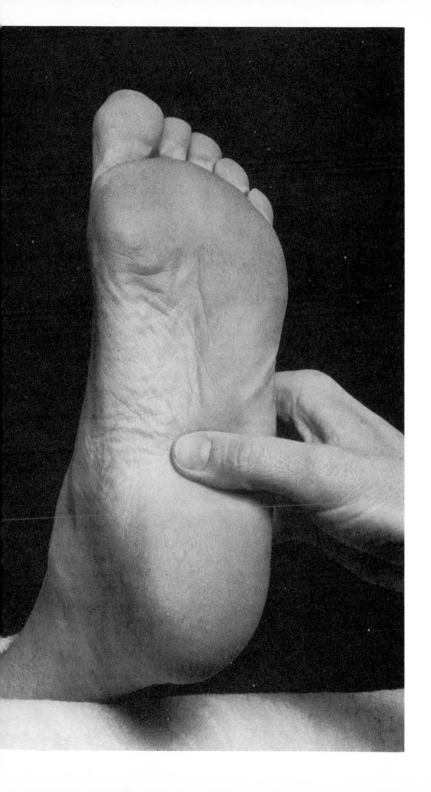

In this photograph the thumb lies across the reflex of the *second horizontal section of the large intestine*. When there is tension, localised contraction can take place, and violent pains can occur, which are known as "spastic colon" pains.

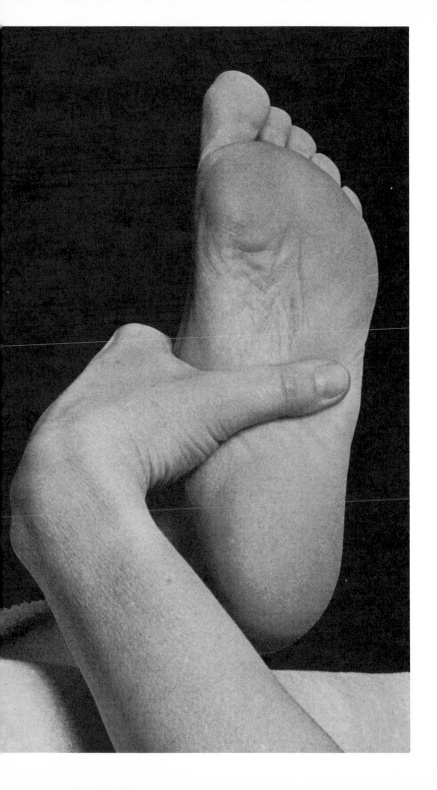

The reflex of the *ileo-caecal junction*. The thumb lies across the transition from the small to the large intestine. If this does not close properly, stomach complaints may result, e.g., excess wind.

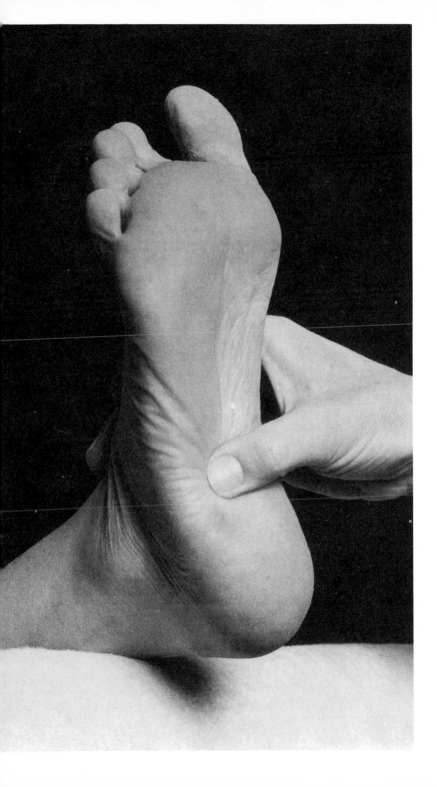

Under the thumb at the level of the nail lies the reflex of the *left kidney* and the *adrenal gland*. In the foot it can be clearly felt like a sort of coffee bean.

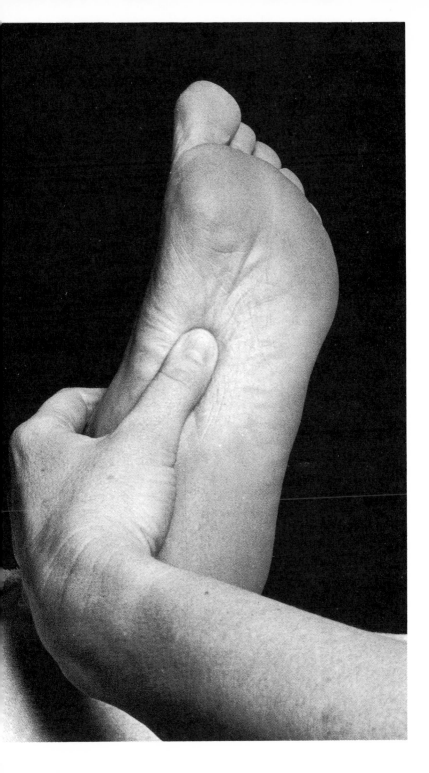

The *bladder* reflex lies inside the circle on the photograph. This is often rather swollen. In the case of a bladder infection, this reflex often turns red.

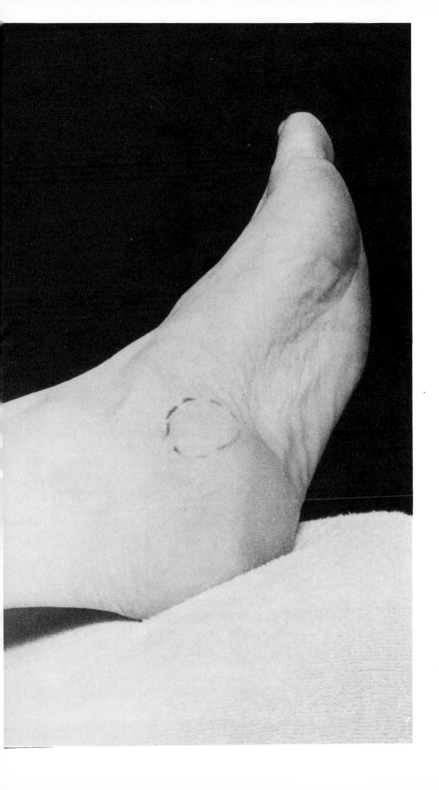

The reflex areas of the *spinal column*. In this photograph the thumb is resting on the reflex of the seventh neck vertebra. The reflexes of the vertebrae are found on the bony edge along the entire inside foot. The muscles are next to these. (See photograph on the following page.)

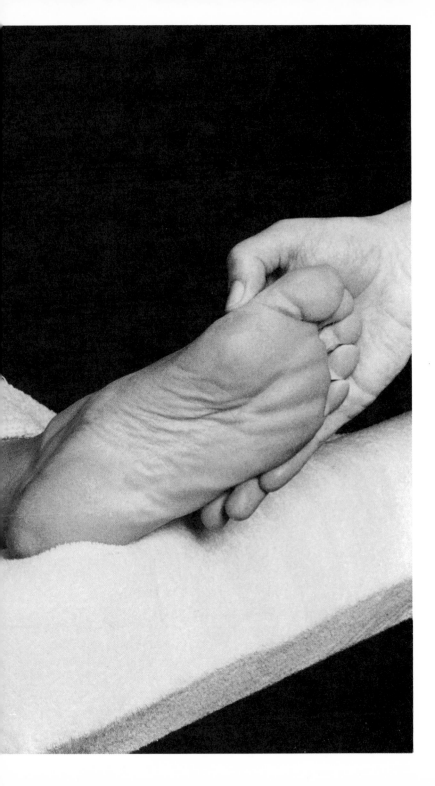

The fingertips in this photograph cover the reflex area of the *lumbar vertebrae*, which is situated above the bladder reflex. There is one thumb's width between them and this area contains the reflexes of the musculature along the lumbar vertebrae.

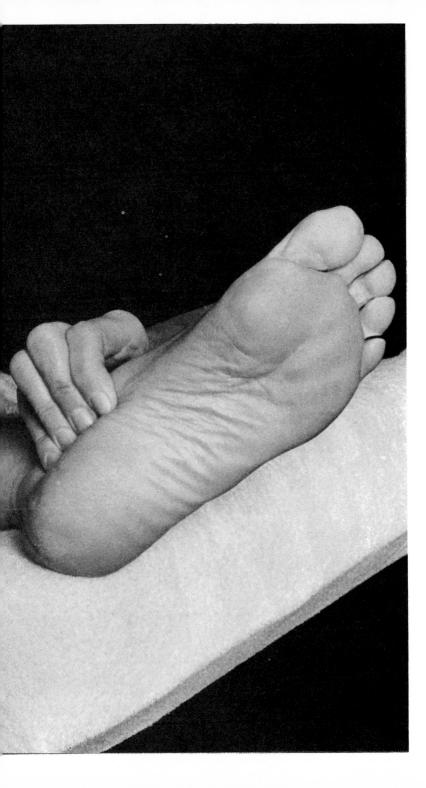

On the heel it is possible to find out from the *sciatic nerve* to
what extent this nerve plays a role in the patient's
complaint.

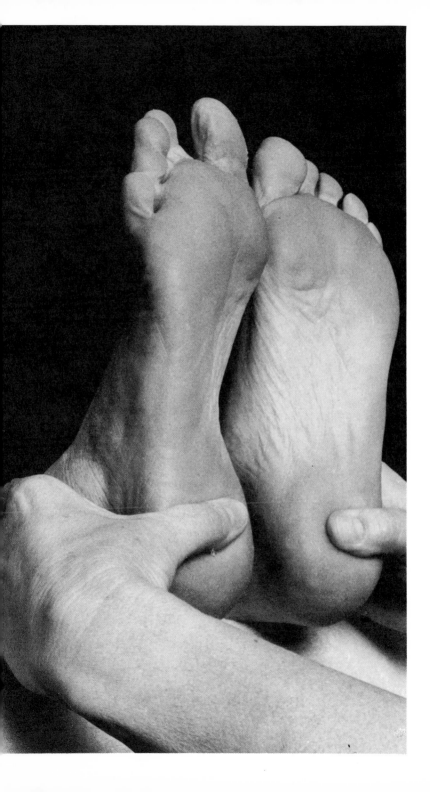

Under the fingernail shown on this photograph lies the reflex of the *uterus* in women and the *prostate* in men. Many menstrual complaints can be prevented by massaging this reflex.

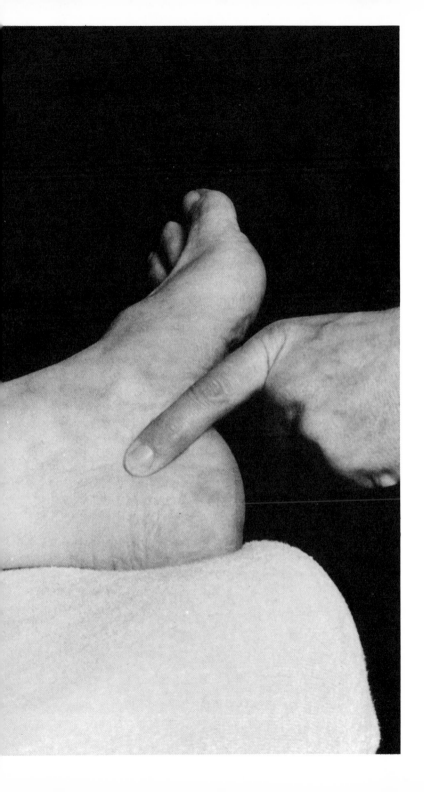

On the side of the outer ankle, just above the reflex area of the muscles of the buttocks, is the reflex of the *testes* in men and the *ovaries* in women. Unlike the reflex of the *uterus/ prostate*, which is rounded, this reflex is elongated.

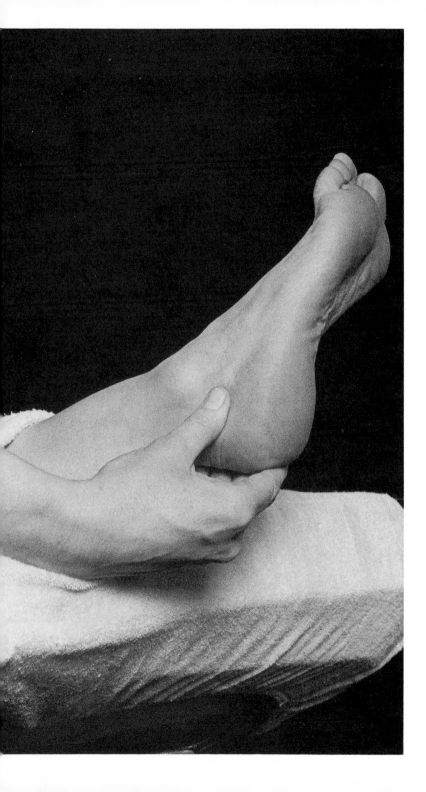

This photograph shows the fingertips on the reflex of the pelvic girdle and the *hips*. The muscles of the buttocks are situated from this point as far as the outer lower edge of the foot. The reflex of the *edge of the hip* lies along the little finger and the ring finger.

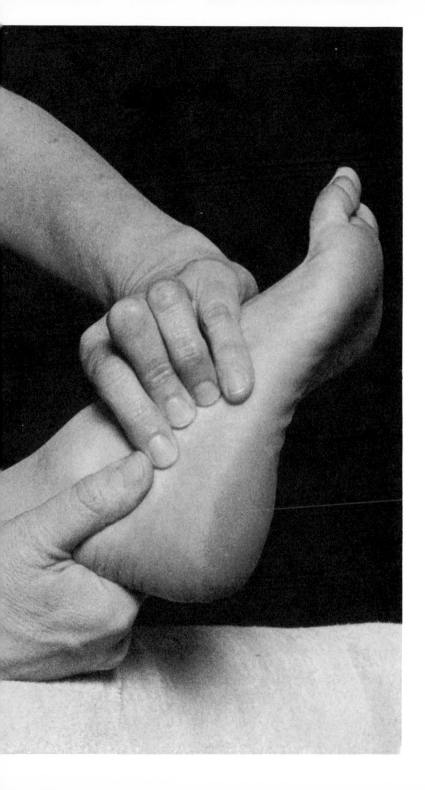

On the side of the pelvis lies the (indirect) reflex of the *knee*, and it is easy to distinguish the bone from the musculature during massage. The *calf* reflex lies a little further down, underneath the foot.

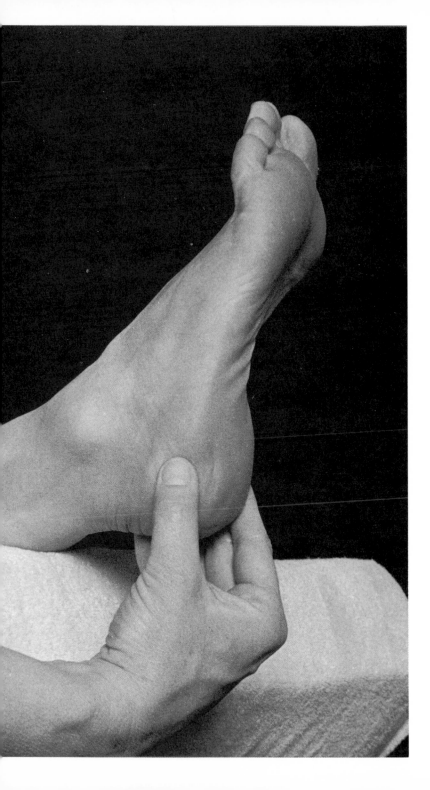

The reflexes of the *lymphatic system* of the lower abdomen and the legs lies around both the inner and outer ankle. In the photograph the thumbs are placed on the reflexes of the *groin*. Swellings of the lymphatic nodes in the groin will be painful when these reflexes are massaged.

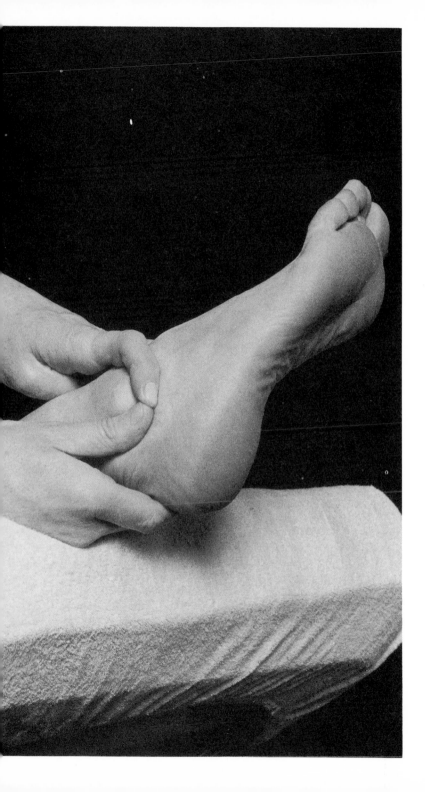

Part V

The projection areas on the foot

Introduction to the massage

Before dealing with the massage of the reflexes themselves, it is necessary to become familiar with some of the basic holds. When you have observed and felt, and possibly smelled the feet, the foot and the lower leg are massaged, using the effleurage technique (stroking).

The ankle joint is gently shaken loose and the end of the foot is rotated from the ankle. These two movements serve to relax the pelvis and the upper abdomen.

Every session of foot massage begins and ends with the *solar plexus*. This important nerve centre lies under the *diaphragm*. Therefore we must begin by locating the position of the diaphragm reflex on the foot. It can be found on a horizontal line below the ball of the foot and on the vertical axis from the middle toe. By pressing with both thumbs on these reflexes *on both feet* at the moment when the patient breathes in, and by releasing at the moment when the patient breathes out, the whole body is relaxed.

It should be noted that any massage carried out in synchronisation with the patient's breathing, will have a more powerful effect.

The zones of the head

Life in the twentieth century requires great powers of endurance and forbearance. Mounting tension is often expressed physically in a series of symptoms starting in the head area. These can be expressed in tense headaches (a feeling of pressure on the head), migraine, problems with sight, dizzy spells, facial pain etc.

Of course, other factors may play a role or be the cause of these complaints. Relaxing the parts of the head suffering from the complaint nearly always gives relief. To achieve this we massage the zones of the head, which are found on the big toe, the four smaller toes and the strip under the four small toes. The sides of the toes are also important because the reflexes of the nerves of the head are situated there. These are usually extremely sensitive on the foot and they often cause a sharp pain. The therapist should take this

Fig. 4 The zones of the head

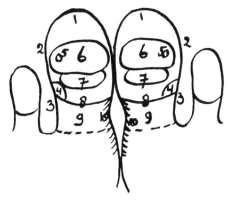

1. dome of the skull; 2. temples; 3. trigeminus (nerve);
4. mastoid; 5. pituitary; 6. cerebral cortex; 7. cerebellum;
8. hairline/base of the skull; 9. neck muscles; 10. vertebrae

possibility into account. Massage of the head area also appears to produce good results in cases of insomnia.

The *pituitary* requires separate treatment. This is the "motor" for a large number of glands which produce internal secretions in our bodies and are responsible for the production of hormones. If any of these glands is defective, this in turn influences the pituitary, and massage of this reflex can have a normalising effect.

Treatment of the *brain* reflexes has a calming and enlightening effect, and this treatment can contribute, inter alia, to:
– Reducing the after-effects of anaesthetics.
– Defects of memory.
– Brain damage.
– Signs of paralysis.

Surprisingly positive results have been achieved by massaging the eye and ear reflexes (blindness, deafness, ear infections.)

Pain can be greatly alleviated by massaging the reflexes of the teeth. Toothache, infected gums, and pain resulting from parts of roots left behind in the gums can be reduced. It goes without saying that bad teeth are, and always will be, the dentist's concern, and that reflexology treatment should certainly not exclude any medical treatment.

Between the area of the zones of the head and the rest of the body there is a transitional area comprising the *neck and shoulder complex*. In addition to pains caused by tension in the neck and shoulders, massage of these reflexes can have an influence on the thyroid and para-thyroid and on the lymphatic system from the arms via the underarm lymph nodes. The thyroid in particular can react very quickly, because this producer of hormones is extremely sensitive to emotion.

The zones of the chest

The organs in the *chest* and the organs high up in the *abdominal cavity* are located in the position of the metatarsals in the foot.

The digestive system can also be found in this area.

On the left foot, the *left lung*, the *heart*, the *spleen* and half of the *stomach* can be distinguished, and directly below the stomach, a large part of the *pancreas*.

The *spleen* is our largest lymph gland. This reflex can be painful on the foot for every form of infection or reduced resistance.

The *lungs* require extra attention for all types of illness related to the air passages, such as, for example, asthma and bronchitis.

The *heart* is an organ which is not normally susceptible to pain during reflexology treatment. However, if the patient is under stress, or is (or has been) over-exerting himself, this reflex may respond painfully because more demands than usual are (or were) made on it. Thus pain in this reflex can serve as a warning to slow down.

Treatment of the heart area is absolutely forbidden immediately after a heart attack, a heart operation, or when the patient has a pacemaker.

The massage can be resumed when the period of convalescence is complete and after the other reflexes are responding normally again.

Foreign bodies can start to "wander" as a result of

reflexology therapy. In this way the object might come to rest in a vital part of the body, with fatal consequences.

The massage can have a disruptive effect for patients with a *pacemaker*. If the heart reflex if left untreated, it is also not possible to treat the left lung for a while, as these two reflexes overlap considerably.

The first part of the stomach comprises an area with a width of two fingers, directly below the joint of the big toe. The *pyloric sphincter* is aptly named, as it is a sphincter. The following rule applies for this area: for malfunctioning of the autonomic nervous system all the reflexes of these sphincters are sensitive. The stomach is a digestive organ, and as such, it soon indicates if there are problems in the system. As is often the case in treatment of the reflex zones, the patient can indicate that he feels a painful reaction in the reflex concerned, without feeling any pain in the organ itself. There is often a lump or hardening in the foot at the point of the stomach reflex, and this shows that the organ is tense. If the patient is not actually experiencing any stomach complaints, it is quite possible that he will feel this tension as a headache or pain in the knee, as explained in the meridian theory mentioned above.

The *pancreas* produces juices which enter the duodenum. The *islets of Langerhans* in the pancreas produce insulin, a hormone which regulates the sugar level in our blood. These glands belong to the group of glands producing internal secretions. Diabetics should only be treated when this can be done in close consultation with the doctor, for it is possible that the patient's functions could become irregular, even though his glands might be functioning better.

The *right lung*, the *liver* with the *gall bladder*, the second part of the *stomach* and part of the *pancreas* are located on the right foot. Through the pyloric sphincter we come to the *duodenum*.

The *liver* has a large number of functions. Detoxification, i.e., checking the blood for harmful components, is very important. It is a large organ, and it takes up a lot of room, both in the body and on the foot.

The *gall bladder* lies under the liver area on a perpendicular line between the third and fourth toe. It plays an important role in the digestion of fats, and in fact, this reflex responds

Fig 5. The zones of the chest

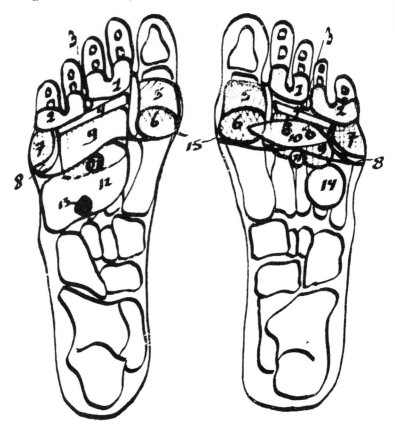

1. eye;   2. ear;   3. inner ear, ringing ears, semicircular canal;   4. pectoral girdle;
5. throat;   6. thyroid and para-thyroid;   7. shoulder;
8. underarm;   9. lung;   10. heart;   10a. heart muscle;
10b. heart valves;   11. solar plexus;   12. liver;   13. gall bladder;   14. spleen;   15. diaphragm.

more sensitively after eating a meal with a high fat content. The liver reflex can also be painful when too many medicines have been taken. Patients suffering from migraine will find that apart from the head zone, the stomach and gall bladder reflexes may also be painful, and not only during a migraine attack. It is well-known that nausea is an important symptom of migraine attacks, and in some cases the patient's vomit may even contain bile.

The pyloric sphincter follows the rule formulated above for sphincters.

The well-known phenomenon of small babies being violently sick is a convulsive reaction of the pyloric sphincter, and this can be successfully relaxed with reflexology. Sometimes small infections occur in the duodenum, particularly when this is one of the patient's weaker organs.

The zones of the abdominal cavity

These are mostly taken up by the *large* and *small intestine*. The reflex of the *appendix* (a worm-like appendage) at the beginning of the vertical section of the colon is also the reflex of the *ileo-caecal junction*, the place which prevents food from returning to the small intestine from the large intestine. When it is tense, this ileo–caecal junction, which is a sphincter, and is controlled by the autonomic nervous system, remains more or less open, resulting in both diahorrea and a great deal of wind. By massaging this reflex it relaxes and functions normally.

In cases of acne it is also possible to treat this sphincter in connection with the lymphatic circulation. In cases of constipation, massaging this reflex can also produce good results.

Internal reflexes are some of the few reflexes that should always be massaged in one direction only, viz., clockwise. If the patient is constipated, the hardness in the reflexes on the feet can be clearly felt and can often be painful during treatment.

The all too familiar painful area of the *spastic colon* (a tensed large intestine) can be found on the left foot next to the last part of the horizontal section of the colon. The large intestine contracts in this place because of nervous tension. The contents of the intestine are crushed together and this results in pain. Malfunctioning of the intestinal system can lead to many problems in the rest of the body.

It is necessary to work very systematically when treating the *urinary system*. To find the *kidneys* one must begin with

Fig. 6. The zones of the abdominal cavity

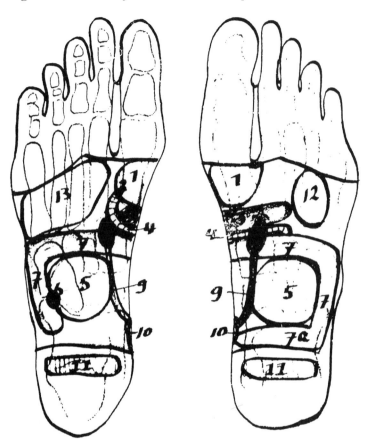

1. stomach;   2. pyloric sphincter;
3. pancreas;   4. duodenum;   5. small intestine;
6. appendix, ileo-caecal junction   7. large intestine;
7a. rectum;   8. kidney and adrenal gland;   9. urethra;
10. bladder;   11. sciatic nerve;   12. spleen;   13. liver;

the *bladder* reflex. The bladder reflex is a swelling on the inside of both feet, which is usually clearly visible and always easy to feel. The reflex lies in the arch under the bony curve on the inside of the feet, slightly in front of the heel and one thumb's width from the bone. The bladder can be visibly large or small, and it is either in its correct position or may have prolapsed to a greater or lesser extent.

Whenever the bladder reflex is no longer on the side of the foot, but has moved inwards to the sole of the foot, this indicates a prolapsed bladder.

In cases of bladder complaints the sphincter muscle is important because of its autonomic nervous function. Bedwetting can be influenced by massaging this reflex (unless there are other causes), and so can incontinence (involuntary loss of urine).

In the following cases, massage of the bladder is advisable: bladder infections, the presence of bladder stones, bedwetting, incontinence, and after operations, if there are problems with urination.

If the big toe is slightly bent backwards, a tendon becomes visible, showing the reflex of the urethra, which lies on the medial side. Following this reflex in the direction of the big toe, you find a slight thickening about the size of a coffee bean: the *kidneys* and the adrenal glands.

The reflex of the kidneys is usually rather sensitive, but when it is out of balance, the pain can be unbearable. The adrenal gland, which is also treated, produces hormones and lies in the upper and outer side of the kidneys. Women in menopause benefit from massage of this reflex because the hormones of the adrenal glands can more or less compensate for the reduced effort of the *ovaries*.

Kidney stones can usually be clearly felt and the patient can certainly feel them on his feet. It is possible to try and break up the kidney stones by using friction. The *sciatic nerve* is found on the part of the sole of the foot that corresponds with the pelvis. This reflex can be treated for both general pain in the lower back and for pain that radiates down the leg (sciatica).

The spinal column

The reflexes of the neck vertebrae are found diagonally against the first joint of the big toe on the medial side. The reflex of the seventh neck vertebra is on the spot where this joint meets the joint of the big toe. This vertebra is found on this joint on the side of the toe. The reflexes of the thoracic vertebrae are positioned exactly along the metatarsal of the big toe. The reflexes of the lumbar vertebrae follow the arch

Fig. 7. The spinal column

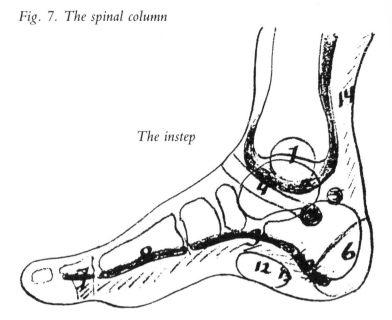

The instep

1. pubis;   2. lymphatic system of the lower abdomen and groin;   3. uterus/prostate;   4. oviduct/sperm duct;
5. anal sphincter;   6. lower pelvis;   7. neck vertebrae;
8. thoracic vertebrae;   9. lumbar vertebrae;   10. sacrum;
11. coccyx;   12. bladder;   13. bladder sphincter;
14. repeat reflex; a. intestines   b. spinal column   c. urogenital zones

of these tarsels, and on the heel they pass into the reflexes of the sacrum, and lastly the coccyx.

Treating these reflexes must be done by placing the thumb against the lower edge of the bone at an angle of 45°. The neural paths radiating from this spinal column are in the same zone, directly against the bony edge, but deeper.

The reflexes of the muscles along the spinal column are in the tissue of the foot at a thumb's width from the bony edge. When these muscles are painful, this tissue in the foot becomes noticeably harder, and this is often visible.

One cannot practise too often on the spinal reflexes in order to learn to distinguish between which vertebrae are, and which are not, how they should be; in this way one can learn to immediately identify any changes in the position of the spine.

In some places along the spinal column one may feel a thickening of the tissue, which can be painful. These correspond to the *plexi*.

The pelvis

If you can imagine recognising a person by his feet, you will certainly understand that the ankle area corresponds to the pelvis, with the upper pelvis on the outside of the feet and the lower pelvis extending a little lower on the inside of the feet.

We will begin with the pelvic area on the *inside of the ankle*.

The ankle bone is the reflex of the *pubis*. If this is wrenched loose in an accident or after a confinement, it is a good idea to treat this reflex to help the healing process.

The reflex of the *prostate* (for men) and *the uterus* (for women) lies in the middle of the line from the ankle to the heel.

It often happens that massage of the prostate reflex helps the prostate to return to its normal size, and in this way it may be able to avoid a prostate operation when this has been thought to be necessary. Massage of this reflex also has a preventative effect because the feet can usually indicate a state of imbalance much sooner than the organ itself, and in this way the massage of the reflex on the foot can prevent problems arising in the organ itself.

The uterus reflex in women is normally more painful than usual just before menstruation, and it is obvious that reflex massage can be used to deal with menstrual complaints.

If the uterus is tilted to the left or right, this can be clearly seen on the foot. The direction of the tilt is shown on the foot by a thickness in the corresponding direction.

During pregnancy the uterus reflex can be massaged normally, unless there have been miscarriages in previous pregnancies.
The use of an i.u.d. means that the uterus reflex should not be massaged.

Fig. 8. The pelvis

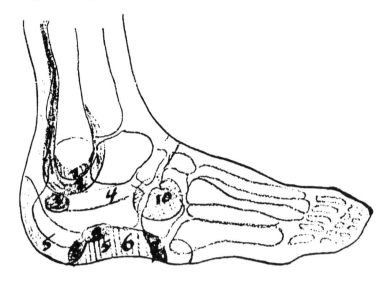

1. hip joint;   2. lymphatic system, lower abdomen and groin;   3. ovaries/testicles;   4. oviduct/sperm duct;   5. upper pelvis;   6. buttock muscles;   7. pelvic girdle;   8. calf;   9. knee;   10. stomach lining

It is extremely possible that the i.u.d. might start to "wander". From the prostate, the sperm ducts, and from the uterus, the oviducts, correspondingly run across the instep to the outside ankle.

Diagonally above the uterus or the prostate respectively, lies the anal sphincter. As this is a sphincter muscle one must remember that it is important for nervous complaints. Massaging this reflex often produces good results in the case of painful haemorroids.

The reflexes of the *testicles* and *ovaries* respectively, are found on the *outside ankle*. The reflexes of the *sperm ducts* and *oviducts* respectively, run along a path which ends below the outer ankle.

The same story applies yet again: the testicles and ovaries are glands which produce internal secretions.

In cases of acne in teenage boys, it is a very good idea to massage this reflex, obviously after first treating the pituitary. In this way the oily secretion of the skin is regulated because the testosterone production is a factor in the excessive secretion of oil. This particular complaint is one that can often successfully be treated with foot massage.

For acne in girls this obviously applies with regard to the ovaries. Similarly, successful results have been achieved in cases where a *testicle* has not dropped properly into the *scrotum*. In this case the massage should be carried out from the testicle reflex, over the foot to the prostate reflex, including the reflexes of the lymphatic system in the lower abdomen (see fig. 8). Massaging the ovaries also produces good results in cases of malfunctions in ovulation (e.g. when a woman stops taking a contraceptive pill), and in cases of cysts.

The lymphatic ducts of the lower abdomen run around the bone of the inner and outer ankle, and can be compared with the groin. In cases where the body retains excessive fluid, these lymphatic ducts can be massaged in order to stimulate the tissue to secrete more fluid. Starting just above the two ankle bones, this reflex lies around them and then goes up about 4 cm. along the Achilles tendon. On either side and immediately next to the Achilles tendon on both feet there are a number of reflexes which seem to repeat the pelvic organs already dealt with earlier, viz., the intestines, the spinal column, the genitalia and the urinary system. In some people these reflexes are extremely painful and consequently the massage must be done carefully so as not to exceed the pain threshold.

The reflex of the *upper pelvis* runs from the top back part of the heel bone, under the reflex of the testicles/ovaries, along the tarsals to the end of the fifth metatarsal. The last part is the reflex of the pelvic girdle.

The semi-circular soft part next to the tarsals is the reflex of the buttock muscles. These can be clearly felt in people after they have been riding or cycling for a day. Unfortunately it is not possible to distinguish between the three different muscles of the buttocks.

The reflexes of the *knee* and *calf* lie on the outside of the foot on the edge of the heel bone. These are known as "indirect" reflexes because they are reflexes of limbs. They are not directly represented on the foot, but are projected onto the pelvic reflex area. In this way they can be massaged normally like direct reflexes. When treating the reflex of the knee it is possible to clearly distinguish the joint and the tendons.

The calf reflex is important in cases of cramp and varicose veins. In cases of cramp in a sportsman, it is easy to notice the difference between the reflex of a cramped leg and that of a normally functioning leg.

Finally there is a spongy swelling which can be seen and/or felt on the upper outer foot. This rather swollen reflex sometimes has a bluish colour and corresponds to all the tissue surrounding the innards, the stomach lining, stomach muscles and skin. This reflex is sensitive after operations on the stomach. It can also indicate that the patient has a paunch. The bluish colour is characteristic of poor circulation.

Organ reflexes on the instep

The reflex area on the middle of the foot, in the first instance corresponds to the ribs. When the pectoral muscles are painful or bruised, e.g., after coughing or sporting accidents, this area should be treated. The layer of tissue is thinner on the top than on the rest of the foot, and the massage should therefore not be so deep. The thumb should not be bent as much, so that the area of contact with the tissue is greater and the pain is therefore more bearable.

The *mammae* (female breasts) are projected onto the rib area. Many women find that their breasts are more sensitive before and during menstruation, and in my experience, this can be prevented in virtually 100% of cases by softly massaging these reflexes before menstruation.

The reflex zone of the *circulation*, and that of the *blood pressure*, as well as all disorders of the blood, such as rheumatism, is found only on the left foot. (The heart reflex lies on the sole of this foot.) People who suffer from cold feet are very sensitive in this reflex. It can be massaged, whether the blood pressure is too high or too low, for the reaction required is to find the balance in the blood pressure. Of course, there may be other physical causes for high blood pressure, which can often also be found on the feet.

The *sternum* can also be found in cross-section opposite

the reflex of the thoracic vertebrae on the side of the first metatarsal, though it ends a little before the ribs.

The reflexes of the *elbow*, the *upper arm* and the *shoulder* are projected on the side of this area corresponding to the ribs.

Fig. 9. Organ reflexes on the instep

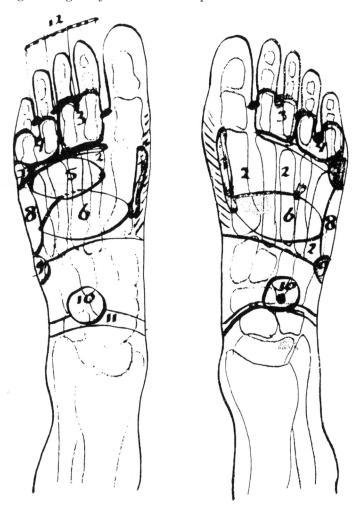

1. sternum;   2. ribs;   3. eye;   4. ear;   5. circulation;
6. female breast;   7. shoulder;   8. upper arm;   9. elbow;
10. stomach wall;   11. oviduct/sperm duct;   12. lymph/
upper abdomen;   13. gall bladder.

In cases of tennis elbow, which actually affects the tendons, the thumb must be moved backwards and forwards around the reflex of the joint as for the knee.

As with the vertebrae, it is possible to distinguish between the reflexes of the bones, muscles and nerves of the upper arm. The shoulder itself has already been covered in the discussion of the shoulder area reflex on the sole of the foot.

The reflex of the *pectoral girdle* can be found on the instep at the joints of the toes. By applying friction to these joints the suppleness or rigidity of the pectoral girdle can be discovered.

For problems with the arms, the neck vertebrae reflex should first be massaged, followed by the neck muscles, the reflexes of the pectoral girdle on both sides of the foot, the upper arm, and finally, the elbow.

The respiratory system

After years of experimentation I have come to an important conclusion regarding our climate. All the reflexes, from the nose to the bronchi, can be found on the big toe and the gap between the big toe and the next toe (see illustration).

If this area is massaged as soon as possible at the onset of a cold, it is possible to prevent the cold taking a grip. If the cold has actually set in, treatment will lead to a rapid response by increased secretion of waste products, which is characterised by mucus production in the nose, sneezing and coughing up phlegm. It is also possible to establish the extent of the cold, whether it is confined to the nose or whether it has spread to the forehead and sinuses, the throat, or even down to the lower respiratory tracts.

Just under the nail of the big toe, but above the joint lying underneath, are the reflexes of the mouth cavity and incisors. This area also covers the gums, the roots of the teeth and the mucus membrane of the mouth.

The reflexes which are massaged to treat pain resulting from gall stones and appendicitis fall outside the description of the foot reflexes. In an acute attack of gall stones the reflex is "trapped" on the foot by placing the thumb on the reflex

Fig. 10. The respiratory system

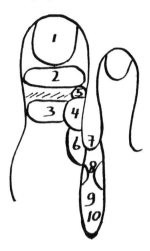

1. scalp;   2. incisors/mouth cavity;   3. nose;   4. jaw
cavity;   5. forehead cavity;   6. tonsils;   7. throat cavity,
also lymph glands;   8. larynx;   9. wind-pipe;
10. bronchi

of the gall bladder and the index finger at right angles to the
foot above the gall bladder reflex (see illustration). This
position is held until the pain in the body subsides.

    The same method is applied in cases of appendicitis, by
placing the thumb on the reflex of the appendix and a finger
at right angles to this in the centre of the stomach areas.

Part VI

An alphabetical list of some common ailments and the method of treatment

1. Abscess
Description:
An accumulation of pus under the skin.
Treatment:
The abscess is brought to a head by careful massage of the reflex of the relevant area.

2. Acne
Description:
The collective term for infections of the sebaceous glands.
Treatment:
Massage of the reflexes of the solar plexus, the digestive organs, the pituitary and the ovaries or testicles, the lymph ducts of the upper and lower abdomen, the liver and the spleen.
Advice: improve through skin care from a beautician.

3. Allergies
Description:
A condition of over-sensitivity to internal or external influences.
Treatment:
Reflex massage of the solar plexus, pituitary and all other glands with internal secretions, lymphatic system and circulation.

4. Back complaints
Treatment:
Reflex massage of the spinal column and the muscles next to it, the pelvis and possibly the stomach and the intestines. Also see nervous tension (stress). Advice on deportment.

5. Bedwetting
Description:
Involuntary urination at night. Can be treated, especially in children.
Treatment:
Reflex massage of the kidneys, (First enquire whether medical supervision is not required.)

6. Bladder infection

Description:
Chronic or acute reaction of the bladder to harmful stimuli.
Treatment:
Reflex massage of the kidneys, urethra and bladder, lymph circulation of the lower abdomen.

7. Bladder, prolapse

Treatment:
Reflex massage of the bladder and sphincter.

8. Breast complaints, pre-menstrual

Description:
Excessive sensitivity of the breasts resulting from swelling of the tissue before menstruation.
Treatment:
Massage the reflexes of the breast twice a week, about ten days before menstruation.

9. Colds

Treatment:
Massage the following reflexes: nose, throat, tonsils, throat cavity, windpipe and lungs, lymph circulation of the upper abdomen, and possibly the reflexes of the eyes and ears.

10. Constipation

Description:
Bowel movement becomes difficult.
Treatment:
Reflex massage of the stomach, large and small intestines, the ilio-caecal junction, the rectum, the lymph circulation of the lower abdomen, repeating the reflex along the Achilles tendon.
Advise on diet, as for haemorroids.

11. Ear disorders

Treatment:
Massage the ear reflexes and lymph circulation of the upper abdomen.

12. Ears, ringing
Treatment:
Massage of ear reflexes and the reflexes of the inner ear.

13. Eye disorders
Treatment:
Reflex massage of the solar plexus, eyes, kidneys and stomach.

14. Haemorroids
Description:
Variscose veins in the anal area.
Treatment:
Massage of the reflex of the anal sphincter, the reflexes of the large and small intestine and the rectum, and the reflex of the lymph circulation in the lower abdomen.
Advise on diet to stimulate peristalsis.

15. Headache
Treatment:
Treat the reflexes of the entire foot and try to ascertain in which organs or systems the cause lies, e.g., hormonal effects, digestion, bile, pectoral girdle, spinal column, eyes, etc.

16. Infertility
Treatment:
Massage the following reflexes: solar plexus, pituitary, ovary, especially between menstruation and ovulation, the oviduct and the uterus, the lower pelvis and the lymph circulation of the lower abdomen.

17. Kidney stones
Description:
Deposits of calcium in the kidneys.
Treatment:
Try to locate the kidney stone on the reflexes and then try to move it from the kidney reflexes towards the bladder via the urethra.

18. Knee complaints
Treatment:
Reflex massage of the pelvis, lymphatic circulation of the lower abdomen, the lower vertebrae and the knee.

19. Legs, cramp in
Description:
Usually involuntary contraction of the muscles accompanied by pain.
Treatment:
Massage of the reflexes of the pelvis, calf, and lymph circulation.

20. Liver disorders
Treatment:
During the period of convalescence from a disease of the liver, it is permissible to massage the reflex of the liver.

21. Menopause
Description:
The complex of physical and psychological factors which accompany the definite end of menstruation.
Treatment:
Reflex massage of the pituitary and adrenal gland. (These often produce a hormone supplement so that the complaint becomes less severe.)

22. Menstrual disorders
Treatment:
A week before menstruation, massage the reflex of the uterus, pelvis, lymph circulation of the lower abdomen, lumbar vertebrae and sacrum.
Two weeks after menstruation: massage the reflexes of the ovaries, the oviduct and the uterus, lymph circulation of the lower abdomen.

23. Migraine

Description:

Headache attacks on one side of the head, which usually last for a few hours, accompanied by nausea and sometimes vomiting.

Treatment:

Treat as for headache. It is important to treat frequently. The migraine can eventually disappear entirely. Initially the migraine attacks may increase, but if the treatment is continued, they will become less frequent and finally they will disappear altogether.

24. Nervous tension/stress

Treatment:

Massage the entire foot rhythmically but not too deeply. Do not give extra massage of the painful reflexes.

25. Oedema

Description:

A build-up of fluid in the deeper layers of the skin.

Treatment:

Reflex massage of the place of swelling, lymph circulation.

26. Pregnancy

Treatment:

Reflex massage of the entire pelvis to stimulate circulation. In this way the pregnancy and the birth will benefit from the improved condition.

27. Ribs, bruises

Treatment:

Locate the reflex position and massage.

28. Scars

Treatment:

Scars often tend to fuse with the underlying tissue. During massage of the corresponding area on the foot they appear as painful and clearly visible lines, swellings or folds. With regular massage two or three times a week for one to four months, good results can be obtained.

Recent scars disappear more quickly than old scars, though the latter can also be removed in the end.

29. Teeth, remains of
Treatment:
Reflex massage of all the teeth.

30. Tennis elbow
Treatment:
Reflex massage of the neck vertebrae and neck muscles, the pectoral girdle, the upper arm and the elbow.

31. Testicles, dropping
Treatment:
Reflex massage of the testes, sperm ducts and the prostate, the lymph circulation of the lower abdomen.

32. Varicose veins
Description:
Dilated twisted blood and/or lymph duct veins, in this case, of the lower leg.
Treatment:
Reflex massage of the calf and lymphatic circulation of the lower leg.